Trauma
An Osteopathic Approach

Jean-Pierre Barral
Alain Croibier

ILLUSTRATIONS BY
Jacques Roth
Alain Croibier

Eastland Press
SEATTLE

Originally published as *Approche ostéopathique du traumatisme*,
Actes graphiques (Saint Étienne), 1997.

English language edition ©1999 by Eastland Press, Inc.
P.O. Box 99749, Seattle, WA 98139 USA
www.eastlandpress.com

ISBN: 978-0-939616-32-9
Library of Congress Control Number: 99-72891

Printed in the United States of America

8   10   9

Book design by Gary Niemeier

Table of Contents

"Only the tissue knows."
—*Rollin Becker*

Foreword

For a very long time I wanted to write a book on the osteopathic approach to trauma. Meeting with Alain Croibier around the time I began this project turned out to be the catalyst.

Alain Croibier is part of the new generation of osteopaths who are setting our science in motion. He and I have known each other for many years and I was fortunate to be his thesis advisor.

His penchant for research, his scientific curiosity, his need for analysis, and his medical knowledge make of him both a teacher and a practitioner of great talent.

While we were practicing in the same region, our ties of friendship and common professional interest were strengthened. In the course of exchanging views and concepts on the means of diminishing the suffering of the too-numerous patients who are victims of trauma, the idea came to us to do this book.

Writing a book "with two pens" is a veritable obstacle course which passion for our profession and friendship helped us to cross with pleasure and calm.

Jean-Pierre Barral

Chapter One:
A Mechanical
Approach to Trauma

Table of Contents

A Mechanical
Approach to Trauma

Introductory Remarks

Trauma can be defined as an injury or wound, whether physical or psychic, caused by an extrinsic agent. In recent years, the desire for a "physical" understanding of bodily trauma has given rise to numerous theoretical and experimental studies. In the attempt to analyze and integrate the mechanisms characteristic of physical trauma, researchers have asked questions such as: How is a bone broken? How much force is required? How is a tissue torn? What happens during avulsion of a tendon? How do tissues react to loads and strains?

Such questions have led to the publication of many works from many different perspectives. In spite of the diversity of opinion, this has ultimately benefited the victims of injury and trauma. Orthopedic surgeons, trauma specialists, and neurosurgeons have been able to establish increasingly effective and specialized treatment protocols for various traumatic injuries.

However, the area of "functional" traumatology remains relatively unexplored. The force of a trauma is frequently insufficient to create a lesion which can be seen with conventional imaging equipment. Because of diffusion of the "principal" trauma, victims often present objective lesions and symptoms which conventional tests do not adequately explain. Such multiple covert lesions or restrictions can be revealed and explained only by manual diagnosis, and properly treated only with a manual approach.

In such cases, what happens to kinetic energy applied to the patient? How do specific tissues incorporate the energy applied to them? What deformations occur during and after the trauma? What are the clinical consequences of trauma? Many of these questions cannot yet be answered conclusively, but certain hypotheses seem more likely than others. We shall describe the many physical parameters which contribute to creation of tissue restrictions before studying them from the osteopathic point of view.

Physical Concepts

The concept of force

"Force" is a basic concept in mechanics. It is difficult to give a precise physical definition. It may be described or understood by the effects it produces: deformation, movement, heat, and friction. Practically speaking, we say that a force has acted on a physical system any time that we observe a change in the state of that system.

> **Classical definition: Force is any agency or influence which changes a body's state of movement or rest.**

Force can also be defined or visualized as the result of interaction between two bodies, either at a distance or through direct contact. Practically speaking, force is a quantity calculated from observable and measurable phenomena. Although it is useful for a mechanistic comprehension of observed phenomena, force is essentially an artificial concept.

Loads and stresses

In mechanics, force can be of external or internal origin.

- Forces of external origin are called *loads* or *applied forces*. Examples: gravity, air resistance, water resistance, muscular action.
- Forces of internal origin are called *stresses*. A stress is the internal resistance of a material subjected to an external load.

Stress can also be defined as the force per unit surface area (e.g., pounds per square inch) exerted when one body pulls on, pushes against, compresses, or twists another body. The concept of stress within a material generalizes the more widely known concept of pressure within a fluid. Since stress is expressed per unit of surface area, it is independent of the overall dimensions of the body in question.

We can consider three principal types of stress *(Fig. 1-1)*.

- Traction (stretching) causes an object to elongate.
- Compression tends to reduce the dimensions of an object.

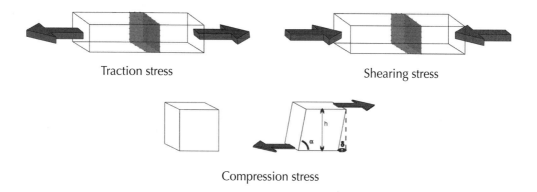

Traction stress

Shearing stress

Compression stress

Fig. 1-1: Different types of stress

• Shearing results from offset forces acting in divergent directions, like scissor blades.

Deformation

Variation in the length of an element which can be stretched or compressed is proportional to its length. Deformation, represented by the symbol ε, is the stretch of the element per unit of length. As the element becomes longer or shorter *(Fig. 1-2)*, the absolute change in its length (L) is referred to as ∅L, and deformation is defined by the equation ε = ∅L / L.

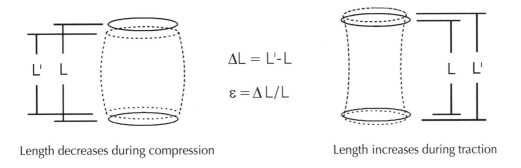

$$\Delta L = L'-L$$

$$\varepsilon = \Delta L/L$$

Length decreases during compression   Length increases during traction

Fig. 1-2: Deformation or relative stretch

Since deformation is the relationship between two lengths, it is a quantity with no units, usually expressed as a percentage. Elastic deformation of common industrial materials is usually less than 0.1%, but certain soft materials such as rubber may stretch by 800%, and some biological tissues even more.

Elasticity, plasticity

Elasticity is the ability of some bodies to regain their shape once the force that deformed them has ceased. Well-known examples of this phenomenon are springs and rubber balls.

Plasticity characterizes the state of a body whose deformations are not reversible. It is the capacity to be deformed in a continuous and permanent manner in one direction, without breaking, in response to a stress greater than the elastic limit.

Relation of stress to deformation

As we apply progressively increasing experimental stress at the edges of a material, the material will stretch and eventually break. By measuring stress and deformation throughout this process, we can construct a graph which is characteristic of the material *(Fig. 1-3)*.

Three distinct areas are seen in this stress-deformation graph:

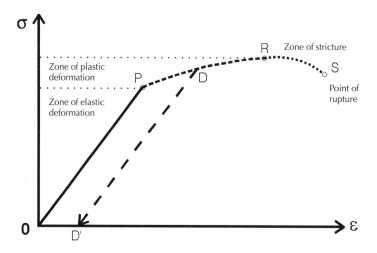

Fig. 1-3: Stress/deformation relationship

ZONE OF ELASTIC DEFORMATION

Stretching (deformation) is proportional to the stress. If the stress is removed, the object regains its initial length; the material is elastic.

ZONE OF PLASTIC DEFORMATION

In this zone, the object does not regain its initial length even if the stress is removed. Some permanent deformation persists, as illustrated by segment DD′ in the figure above. Point P indicates the transition from elastic to plastic deformation.

ZONE OF STRICTURE AND BREAKAGE

Beyond point R, further increase of stress does not result in continued deformation; the material has reached its limit of plasticity. Soon thereafter, the material reaches its breaking point (S).

Energy of deformation

During deformation of an elastic material, it stores energy which is released when the stress is removed. The quantity of energy released may be considerable. For a material which is completely elastic, stored energy W (expressed in joules) resulting from stress producing deformation is given by the formula: $W = \frac{1}{2}\varepsilon\sigma$ *(Fig. 1-4).*

During a traumatic event, a significant quantity of kinetic energy is applied to the body and transmitted or "injected" over a very short period of time into various tissues which are heterogeneous, anisotropic (showing different responses along different axes), and show various degrees of elasticity. Only a part of this energy results in deformation. Another part is dispersed as heat. The remaining part is stored in the tissues as residual energy, which may persist for a surprisingly long time. For example, we have cases in which a spleen ruptures up to forty days after a traumatic event.

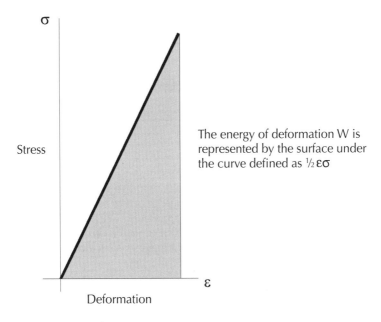

The energy of deformation W is represented by the surface under the curve defined as $\frac{1}{2}\varepsilon\sigma$

Fig. 1-4: Energy of deformation

Mechanics of Trauma

The term "trauma" refers in a general way to all bodily lesions resulting from any form of external assault. This often involves kinetic energy leading to a mechanical injury. However, the concept of trauma can be extended to other thermal, chemical, physical, or mechanical phenomena which cause injury. The term "psychic trauma" refers to psychological manifestations which follow a traumatic event.

Principal agents of trauma

There are many types of trauma *(Table 1-1)*. Traumas due to mechanical assault are the most frequently encountered in our practice, and are discussed in detail below.

Definition of lesions

Traumatic lesions are defined by the mode of application and dissipation of the physical energy released during the very short duration of an accident (as little as 50 milliseconds), and by the mechanical characteristics of the bodily structures involved.

At the time of the accident, the physical forces set in motion determine the *immediate lesions*. The nature and importance of these lesions are dictated by the circumstances of the accident and the size of the forces. Traumatic lesions produced in this way are progressive. During subsequent hours and days, dynamic phenomena take place and cause *secondary* or *late lesions*. Finally, after gradual healing (with or without treatment), some lesions persist with varying degrees of pathology which constitute the *sequelae*.

Type of trauma	Mechanism of lesion	
Mechanical Action	• Impact against an obstacle from projection or a fall • Impact from a falling object or crushing • Phenomena of inertia due to sudden acceleration or deceleration • Penetrating wound from gun or object; in the extreme, traumatic amputation	
Physical Action	• Blast injury from vibration • Crush syndrome from compression, without crushing • Accidents involving decompression in water or air	
Thermal Action	*Burns*	• From radiation • From contact with a very hot substance • From Joule effect of an electric current
	Frostbite	• From refrigeration (0 to -4°) • From freezing (< to -4°)
Chemical Action	• Necrobiosis from acids or bases • Poisoning	

Table 1-1: Classification of trauma according to causal agent (after PATEL)

CLASSIFICATION OF LESIONS

Contusions are closed lesions resulting from direct impact, that is, the projection of an object traveling at high speed on a fixed body. The severity depends on the intensity of impact and the region affected. We speak of contusions of the soft tissues (skin, fascia, muscle), osseous contusions, cartilaginous contusions, and so on.

Wounds result from the impact of a cutting or perforating object which breaches the body covering (skin). The severity depends upon extent, depth, and, above all, location of the impact.

Osteoarticular lesions are named after the tissue specifically injured: the skeletal system and joints.

- *Sprains* are simple lesions due to fascial or ligamentous injury.

- *Dislocations* represent partial or total separation of the joint surfaces and are often accompanied by ligamentous injury.

- *Fractures* involve a "dissolution of continuity" in the bone. The fracture may be open or closed, depending upon whether there is associated injury to the skin. Fractures and dislocations result from varied mechanisms (direct impact, torsion, tearing, compression stress, flexion, traction), the study of which falls outside the scope of this book.

Crushing is associated with other lesions such as fractures or wounds, and occurs during accidents in which a part of the body is subjected to significant pressure. Its severity depends on the topography of the affected area and the magnitude of the pressure and other forces involved.

Amputations are complete separations of some part of the body, usually a limb. There are different types, depending upon the nature of the initial accident, for example, complete section or tearing.

Types of mechanical trauma

As osteopaths, we view trauma primarily as a mechanical event. There are two major types of mechanical trauma: related to contact and related to inertia. Both types can be reproduced experimentally or observed in isolation in clinical practice. However, the majority of cases that we see, particularly traffic accidents, involve both types simultaneously.

- *Effects of contact* are observed any time the body hits or is hit by an object. Lesions occur not only locally at the point of impact, but also at distant sites as a result of shock waves and similar phenomena.
- *Effects of inertia* are observed when the body is subjected to acceleration and/or deceleration. Most often this affects the skull and vertebrae, as in whiplash. Lesions are diffuse and often multifocal.

Experimental studies of trauma

Many laboratories have attempted to study the effects of trauma on animals by *in vivo* or post mortem experiments. The object is to gain better understanding of the results of trauma in humans by extrapolating the results. However, because there are so many variable parameters in a living person, such experiments have had limited usefulness.

It is often stated that the human body is composed of 206 bones. More importantly, it is composed of billions of cells, all of which are capable of being injured during an accident. The experimental studies with which we are familiar point to the existence of *global lesions* which may be far removed from the symptom. This concept of the global lesion is at the foundation of osteopathy. It reflects our belief that nothing is isolated in a living organism and that all structures and processes are interdependent. Clinically, this concept leads us to treat people instead of symptoms, and to look at the entire person and his bodily structure, instead of simply the place that hurts.

In the 1980s, the French National Institute for Research on Transportation and Safety (INRETS) performed experiments with 30 pigs, some anesthetized and some awake, secured in automobiles (Verriest, 1986). The pigs were thrown against a wall in cars going at speeds from 10 to 55 km/h, with accelerations of 10 to 25 g in 50 milliseconds. Speed and deceleration were both significant determinants of trauma. In other experiments with monkeys, the cranium was removed and intracranial pressure sensors were placed and covered with glass.

Such experiments have been discontinued (to the great relief of the many people opposed to research using live animals) in favor of studies using lifelike mannequins or cadavers. However, the absence of all cerebral and even unconscious psychological activity, metabolism, tone, and modification of tissue viscoelasticity in the cadaver studies render the interpretation and significance of their results questionable at best. In view of the limitations of the above studies, we prefer to select and review certain physical laws which have enhanced our clinical understanding of trauma and its effects.

Physical laws related to mechanical lesions

Acceleration, deceleration, and inertia

Most traumatic accidents involve movements which are accelerated rather than uniform. In physics, *acceleration* is defined as the change in velocity per unit time. Acceleration may be positive (speed increasing during the interval of time in question), zero (speed remaining constant over time), or negative (speed decreasing over time) *(Fig. 1-5)*.

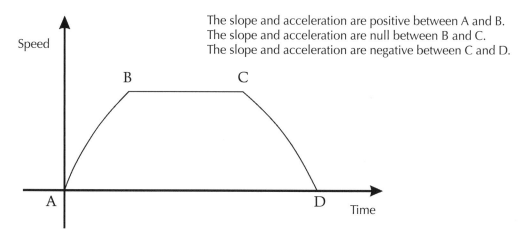

Fig. 1-5: Graph of the speed of an automobile as a function of time

Negative acceleration is usually referred to as *deceleration (Fig. 1-6)*. In principle, acceleration and deceleration have equal pathogenic potential.

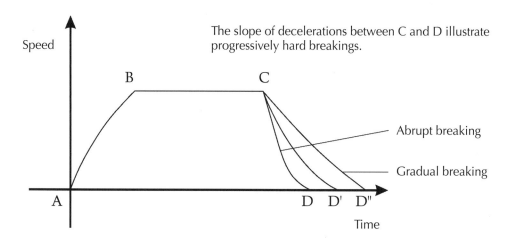

Fig. 1-6: Slope of breaking and deceleration

Velocity is measured in meters per second and time is measured in seconds; acceleration is expressed in meters per second per second (abbreviated as m/s², or "meters per second squared"). An average acceleration of 1m/s² corresponds to an average increase in speed of 1m/s per second.

Effects of inertia occur any time that a trauma directly or indirectly produces acceleration or deceleration of all or part of the body. Consider the head, which can be accelerated by a blow setting it in motion and decelerated abruptly by an obstacle interrupting its movement. We will refer to such events as *shock* and *aftershock*.

Similarly, backward impact in a vehicle standing still will cause rapid acceleration of the occupant's craniocervical segment in the direction of extension, and the deceleration immediately following will occur in the direction of flexion of the cervical spine.

Several types of acceleration may be distinguished, as follows.

LINEAR ACCELERATION

An idealized concept, linear acceleration describes a unidirectional trajectory of impact. Even if we claim that an impact is unidirectional, we know that the shock wave is never linear, because of different qualities and densities of tissues. Authors who focus on the head and neck consider acceleration to be linear if the head remains within the axis of the body.

ANGULAR ACCELERATION

Angular acceleration relates to a curve-shaped trajectory of the head upon impact, and associated shearing forces. Angular acceleration of the head plays an important role in lesions of the skull tissues. The craniospinal angle modifies the amplitude of the impact during trauma.

WEIGHT ACCELERATION

From a mechanical point of view, weight (or mass) is one of the factors which most influences the human body, because we deal constantly with the force of gravity. Falling objects undergo acceleration because of their weight: *the force of gravity or gravitational attraction* exerted by the earth. Acceleration of an object near the earth's surface is represented by the value g, which is approximately 9.8m/s². Speed of a falling object at the moment of impact increases with distance fallen.

The value g is often used as a comparative unit in a "scale of acceleration." We say, for example, that a Formula One driver gains 3 g in the turns, or that a fighter pilot gains 20 g during ejection. This signifies that the acceleration in these situations is respectively three or twenty times that of the person's normal weight acceleration. During acceleration, the race car driver or pilot subjectively feels his weight increase to the level of normal weight multiplied by the number of g *(Table 1-2)*.

PHYSIOLOGICAL EFFECTS OF ACCELERATION

Developments in supersonic aviation and space exploration have stimulated much research into the effects of acceleration on the human body. More mundanely, all of us have experienced such effects (particularly abdominal sensations) in response to vertical acceleration in an elevator, horseback riding, merry-go-round, and the like.

Type of acceleration	Acceleration (expressed in g)	Duration (seconds)
Elevators		
Express	0.1–0.2	1–5
Comfortable limit	0.3	
Emergency stop	2.5	
Automobile		
Comfortable stop	0.25	5–8
Very uncomfortable stop	0.45	3–5
Quickest possible stop	0.70	3
Accident (survival possible)	20–100	0.05–0.1
Airplane		
Normal take-off	0.5	10–20
Catapult take-off	2.5–6	1.5
Disaster landing (survival possible)	20–100	
Ejectable seat	10–23	0.25
Falling		
Opening of parachute	8–33	0.2–0.5
Parachute landing	3–4	0.1–0.2
Fall in fireman's net	20	0.1

Table 1-2: Approximate duration and order of magnitude of several brief accelerations (after Kane & Sternheim)

These effects are related to two factors: (i) the heterogeneity of solid and fluid structures within the human body; (ii) inertia promoted by the elastic compartments in which the fluid structures circulate or reside.

When our bodies accelerate upward, blood and fluids accumulate in the lower part of the body (positive g). Conversely, when the acceleration is downward, the volume of blood and fluids increases in the upper part of the body (negative g). The abdominal viscera comprise a semi-fluid mass which responds to upward or downward acceleration in a similar manner, often to our distress.

One's resistance to acceleration depends upon the degree and duration of the acceleration. Because of the inertia of bodily liquids and elasticity of the organs, the effects of moderate acceleration (up to several g) are minor if the acceleration lasts only a fraction of a second. The tolerance limit for brief acceleration is several dozen g; it is determined by structural resistance of the vertebra and skeletal system. The longer the acceleration lasts, the greater the risk of tissue or skeletal damage.

Studies of people such as the aforementioned race car driver or pilot who encounter prolonged, intense acceleration reveal characteristic circulatory problems. Two well-known examples are:

- at 3 g: visual distortion due to lack of oxygen in the retina
- at 6 g: loss of consciousness due to decrease of cerebral blood flow.

Through a combination of physical training, pilot's position, contraction of abdominal muscles, and pressurized flight cabin, the human tolerance limit may be pushed past 9 or 10 g.

During trauma from inertia or impact, the effects of acceleration are considerable. Kinetic energy and the force of inertia subject the components of the body to a difficult test. Even if compensating neuromuscular circuits are not activated by an unexpected blow, fascial and ligamentous structures which support inertia and oppose movement during the shock and aftershock are activated. The attachment system for each visceral organ or other body structure was designed to resist normal forces. However, nothing in human evolutionary history prepared us for the very large forces that appear during such uniquely modern traumas as motor vehicle accidents. It is not surprising that such accidents can produce many deleterious effects.

Problems caused by acceleration are usually lesions due to stretching and elongation of connective tissue structures. Different degrees of stretching may be noted, from limited stretching to breakage or osseous tearing at insertion sites. The familiar cervical sprain is an example. It is characterized by distention or rupture of the intervertebral ligaments on a particular level.

Weight and mass

Technically, the weight of an object (W) represents gravitational force (g) acting upon the mass (m) of the object. The mass of an object is a constant, determined by the quantity of matter contained in the object. It is the same if the object is in Paris, on the moon, or in space. The weight of an object, in contrast, varies depending on location and represents the force of attraction by gravity at that location: W = m g.

ACTUAL WEIGHT

The weight which we perceive under given conditions is determined by forces exerted by the earth or what supports us. Actual weight is zero for a person in free fall. During significant acceleration, actual weight may be much greater than real weight. This phenomenon is put to use in the laboratory, where centrifuges increase the actual weight of certain cellular components in order to increase their separation. Ultracentrifuges can attain accelerations of 500,000 g.

Of more everyday relevance to us, when an elevator goes up, it begins by accelerating and then attains a constant speed which it maintains until it decelerates in order to stop. During upward acceleration, we feel heavier than usual. When the elevator descends, we feel lighter than usual.

Actual weight is defined as the total force that a person or object exerts on a scale. If some acceleration force (a) other than gravity (e.g., an elevator) is affecting the person, the formula W = m g can be modified to W_{actual} = m ($g + a$) or m ($g - a$), depending on whether the other force is acting in the same direction as gravity or the opposite direction.

The concept of weight depending on acceleration is necessary to understand trauma-related lesions. As shown in the examples above, a person's actual weight is directly related to the number of g to which she is subjected. Imagine what happens to a vertebral body or intervertebral disk subjected to a load 20, 50, or 100 times greater than normal!

This concept applies to both visceral and neurological components of the body. During traumatic acceleration, the effective weight of these components inside their cavities increases greatly. This overload may occur in directions which are neither habitual nor physiological. Many structures of support and maintenance may be constrained or stretched, creating tissue stretching with reactive irritation. Body fluids are similarly affected by increases in actual weight.

Collisions and energy

Definition of energy

According to modern physics, everything is energy. The human body represents an extremely evolved form of organized matter. Our cells, body fluids, and tissues comprise a specific organization of elementary molecules and atoms, primarily carbon, oxygen, and hydrogen. Quantum physics teaches us that these atoms themselves constitute a particular level of organization of small *quanta of energy*. We conclude that a human being represents a highly evolved form of energy organization.

The concept of energy plays a fundamental role in many branches of physics, and has a variety of definitions. In mechanics, energy is usually defined as *the capacity to perform work*. When an object is capable of exerting force over some distance, it has energy. Energy can exist in different forms, including heat, light, and electricity.

Forms of mechanical energy

Mechanical work can be considered as the product of a force and a displacement. A mechanical system capable of performing work contains "work in reserve" or energy. This energy is called:

- *potential energy* if due to the spatial position of the constituents of the system
- *kinetic energy* if the body is moving.

POTENTIAL ENERGY

We speak of potential energy (PE) when we want to associate the position of a body with its capacity to perform work. For example, a person who weighs 50kg and is 2m above the ground has potential energy relative to the ground. PE in this situation is equal to the work required to lift the weight from the ground to the defined position. The person possesses 1000 J of potential energy, calculated as the product of force times height: $PE = F h = m g h$.

KINETIC ENERGY

The kinetic energy (KE) of an object reflects the work that the object can achieve through its movement. Kinetic energy of an object of mass m traveling at speed v is defined as $KE = \frac{1}{2} mv^2$.

A fundamental principle of physics is that the final kinetic energy of an object is equal to its initial kinetic energy, increased by the total work performed by all the forces exerted upon this object *(Fig. 1-7)*.

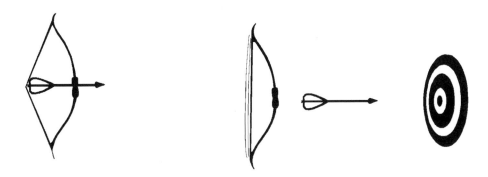

The work provided to bend the string is stored in the form of potential energy.

This liberated energy is transformed into the kinetic energy of the arrow.

Fig. **1-7:** Potential energy and kinetic energy

Law of conservation of mechanical energy

The law of conservation of energy dominates physics, and we can observe it in purely mechanical phenomena. In the absence of friction and heat, total mechanical energy, which equals the sum of potential and kinetic energy, remains constant, although one term may increase as the other decreases. This is the principle of the conservation of mechanical energy.

In many cases, dissipative forces transform mechanical energy into other forms of energy, such as the heat and noise produced by a saw or drill. Heat represents energy which has been transferred to the molecules which constitute the substance. This transfer of energy increases the average speed of the molecules, that is, their thermal energy.

Laws of collisions

In the physical sense, a collision consolidates all the "contact" phenomena between two material points. The important aspect of the phenomenon resides in the slight duration of contact relative to duration of the displacements observed. The integral of the force of a collision over its duration constitutes impulse.

Elastic and inelastic collisions

During a collision, the total quantity of energy is conserved, but kinetic energy is not necessarily conserved. For example, when a rubber ball is dropped on the ground, it bounces back to a height almost equal to its initial one. The quantity of mechanical energy dissipated when the ball touches the ground does not matter. If, however, a ball of putty falls, it remains on the ground because all its kinetic energy is either dissipated in the form of heat or used during the work of deformation *(Fig. 1-8)*.

A collision in which mechanical energy is conserved is termed an *elastic collision*. When mechanical energy is not conserved, the collision is *inelastic*. During a totally inelastic collision (the ball of putty example), relative movement ceases. The

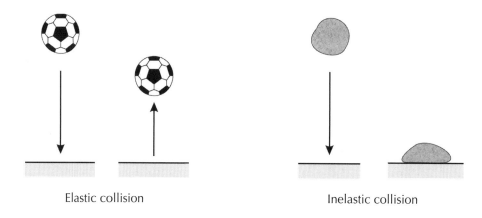

Elastic collision   Inelastic collision

Fig. 1-8: The two types of collision

quantity of energy dissipated in the form of heat or work of deformation of objects depends upon their relative mass.

When the mass of the moving object is small relative to the mass of the stationary object, most of the kinetic energy is lost during the collision and the final kinetic energy is small.

LAW OF CONSERVATION OF TOTAL ENERGY

Conservation of energy is a fundamental and general concept with applications to biological, mechanical, chemical, meteorological, astronomical, and many other processes.

Energy is manifested in many forms. If we calculate or measure total energy (i.e., the sum of mechanical, electrical, thermal, and other energies) before and after some dynamic process, we find that total energy remains constant even if a particular form of energy is not conserved. Although energy can be transformed from one form to another, it is never created or destroyed.

This is the principle of *conservation of total energy*.

Historically, it has been noted that at times when the principle of the conservation of energy seemed not to apply, a new form of energy was about to be identified. The law of conservation of total energy was not completely understood until Einstein demonstrated the relationship between matter and energy. He proved not only that energy can be transformed from one form to another, but also that energy can be transformed into matter and vice versa.

Whereas total energy is always conserved, mechanical energy is often converted to other forms. In this book, we deal with traumatic events that begin with mechanical energy. How can the diverse energies which follow trauma be expressed? What happens to the energy that is not used in the work of deformation? How do the tissues receive and tolerate the quantity of energy applied to them during trauma?

Momentum and impulse

These concepts are useful for understanding the effect of a force during a brief period, such as during a collision. In daily life, many phenomena can be viewed as collisions, even though we may not think of them this way, for example, being punched on the shoulder, jamming on the brakes of a car, being a passenger with seatbelt fastened during an automobile accident, running, or falling on the ground.

MOMENTUM

The *momentum* of an object is defined as the product of its mass times its linear velocity: $p = m\ v$. The international scientific unit for momentum is the kilogram-meter per second. When two objects collide, the momentum of each changes, but the total momentum of the system is conserved.

IMPULSE

An external force will alter the momentum of a body. Depending on the direction of the force, momentum will increase or decrease. The important parameters determining the change of momentum are the magnitude and duration of the applied force.

Impulse is defined as the product of the average force multiplied by the time over which it acts on a body: $dI = F\varnothing t$, and is measured in newton-seconds (Ns). It equals the change or variation of momentum of the body.

For example, momentum is increased in sports such as throwing or jumping by applying a force for a long period of time. On the other hand, in sports such as tennis, baseball, golf, or hockey, where impact with the ball or puck is brief, a strong force is needed to significantly increase momentum.

The impulse needed to stop an object corresponds to the object's initial momentum. If braking occurs over a long period, the force needed is less than if it occurs over a short period.

The concept of impulse is also illustrated when a ball hits a tennis player with great force. If the ball hits a part of the body in which the bones are subcutaneous (tibia, greater trochanter, skull), the change in momentum (impulse) is much more sudden than if it hits soft tissue (abdomen, thigh, shoulder). The ball exerts weaker force in the latter case.

This principle explains why falling from even a low height may be dangerous if one falls on a part of the body which is incapable of absorbing impact.

APPLICATION TO TRAUMA

When trauma occurs over a long duration, the body has time to bring its compensatory mechanisms into play. The shorter the duration of impact, the greater the impulse, and the greater the likelihood of lesions. The duration of traumatic events is typically 50 to 90 milliseconds. This is too short for the compensatory mechanisms, and therefore may result in lesions. The principle can be illustrated with an example *(Fig. 1-9)*.

Suppose that a man weighing 100kg, with a center of mass one meter above the ground, falls on his hip after hitting an obstacle.

- If the collision lasts 0.1 second, the ground exerts a force of 4200 newtons on his hip, which is sufficient to cause a fracture.
- If the collision lasts for one second, the ground exerts a force of only 420 newtons, which most often causes only a bruise.

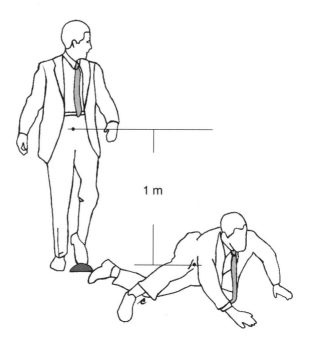

Fig. 1-9: Fall on a hip (after Williams, Lisner & Le Veau)

When falling or jumping, a person can increase the time before they hit the ground. The force can be reduced by changing the angular momentum through bending of the ankles, knees, and hips, or curling into a ball. According to Benedek and Villars (1973), "One can fracture the bones in one's leg or ankle by jumping in a contracted or crumpled fashion with the joints rigid even from a height as low as two meters."

In general, increasing collision time decreases the risk of injury. This can be achieved by making floors and walls out of more flexible materials, wearing a helmet, or similar measures.

Shock wave

In physics, a "shock wave" is generated when a moving object travels faster than the propagation speed of the wave it causes in its medium. Spherical waves previously emitted by the source are tangent to the cone of revolution whose axis is the rectilinear trajectory of the source. The cone, surrounded by the spherical waves emitted, progresses with the source and constitutes the shock wave. This phenomenon is easily observable in two dimensions in the movement of a boat in calm water; the greater the speed of the boat, the smaller the angle at the top of the cone *(Fig. 1-10)*.

Application of this idealized model to the human body is problematic at best. Even if transmission of a shock wave to a homogeneous environment can be analyzed, the heterogeneity of body tissues greatly complicates analysis.

An important point is that vibrations and shock waves are transmitted best by dense media. The harder the substance, the more directly the waves are transmitted. In the body, bones and hard organs are the best vectors of shock waves, but liquid-filled compartments can also transmit them fairly well.

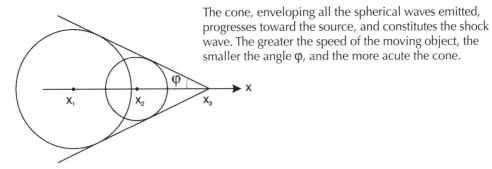

The cone, enveloping all the spherical waves emitted, progresses toward the source, and constitutes the shock wave. The greater the speed of the moving object, the smaller the angle φ, and the more acute the cone.

Fig. 1-10: Shock wave caused by a moving object

Fragile "reservoir organs" such as the spleen may break when the body is subjected to violent trauma, even if the point of impact is not in the organ's immediate vicinity. Likewise, fractures may occur opposite the point of impact, where the shock wave has focused the energy of collision.

Energy transfer

Our colleague Pierre Tricot (1992) mentions three major methods for the transfer of energy.

FLOW

Energy travels from one point to another in the form of a wave with defined wavelength and frequency.

IMPLOSION/ EXPLOSION

Energy is propagated in all directions relative to a given point. Movement is centrifugal (i.e., goes outward in all directions) in explosions, and goes inward from all directions toward the point in implosions. Geometrically, explosion and implosion can be considered as multidirectional energy flow propagated toward or from an epicenter.

BLOCKED FLOW

Blocked flow fails to circulate normally because it is blocked either by an obstacle or by one or several flows in the opposite direction. The pressure of running water in pipes illustrates this concept. While the tap is closed, the energy from the water pressure is contained in the pipe. As soon as the tap or valve is opened, the water can flow out.

ENTRY AND EXIT OF THE ENERGY OF COLLISION

During impact, the energy of collision produces primarily deformation of the body, expressed by movement and perhaps by heat. When quantity of energy of collision is moderate, the most frequent result is a contusion.

With greater force, deformation can lead to gradual bone displacement, subluxation, or even dislocation. In situations in which the stress has no outlet in the joint mechanics, fractures may occur.

During a blow, surrounding tissues are theoretically deformed with projection perpendicular to the direction of impact. The cranial cavity is deformed due to osseous elasticity and suture lines, as much as one centimeter in the transverse direction! Intracranial elements are affected by movement of the cervical spine which deforms the cranial cavity, causing excessive intracranial pressure which can lead to further deformation. The increased intracranial pressure has repercussions throughout the spinal canal. This phenomenon also explains why the posterior part of the brain tends to be pushed toward the foramen magnum. It is easy to imagine that excessive pressure affects all the obstacles surrounding the cord, including both natural anatomic obstacles and acquired ones, such as arthritis.

This explains why the *prelesional state* is important. Many patients who present with asymptomatic arthritis experience severe pain after minimal trauma, due to the prelesional state. Even if there is only one significant restriction in the prelesional state, the forces of collision cannot be distributed and dampened normally. They converge where mobility and capability of distention are smallest.

In conclusion, any osseous irregularity or tissue restriction can serve to focus lesions. For example, Goldsmith (1966) demonstrated that with identical values of acceleration, excess cranial pressure is inversely proportional to the internal diameter of the skull. Statham (in Gurdjian and Webster, 1958) noted that, in dogs, acceleration is always accompanied by an increase in intracranial pressure.

ACCUMULATION AND SATURATION OF ENERGY

The concept of the accumulation and saturation of energy in specific body areas is difficult to prove. A certain quantity of kinetic energy is applied to the body during trauma. The body must absorb this energy, which is transformed in the tissues, primarily in the form of heat and deformation. Fractures, ruptures, and dislocations represent conversion of kinetic energy into the work of deformation.

However, all the kinetic energy may not be channeled into these major lesions. According to the law of conservation of energy, the quantity of kinetic energy unused by the work of deformation will be converted into potential energy.

This potential energy is apparently stored in soft tissues, primarily elastic connective tissues. Because of their elasticity, these tissues are capable of significant deformation, some by as much as 800%. However, above a certain deformation threshold, they may no longer be able to regain their original mechanical characteristics. Thus, certain body areas challenged by one or more traumas can retain some quantity of energy of traumatic origin.

Changes in pressure and cavitation

During trauma, intracavity pressure is modified. Pressure differentials have been extensively studied in the brain. Because of differences in their density, the brain and skull react very differently to impact. Displacement of the brain mass in the direction of the osseous wall causes change in pressure, which can produce "cavitation bubbles" capable of creating cerebral microlesions.

According to Goldsmith, trauma produces pressure gradients in all fluids except gelatin. The phenomenon of cavitation exists in all fluids, and is recognized by osteopaths in the synovial fluid. Goldsmith believes that cavitation occurs in cerebral fluids such as blood and cerebrospinal fluid, but not in the cerebral tissue itself (Goldsmith, 1966).

In addition to cavitation, pressure gradients play a role in formation of lesions. Differences in pressure are compensated for by the cerebrospinal fluid, intracranial membranes, foramen magnum, ear drums, internal auditory canals, eyeballs, and the numerous foramina at the base of the skull. In the pelvis a corresponding role is played by the obturator foramina and all the natural orifices. In the thorax, pressure compensation ("dampening") occurs at the intercostal spaces, diaphragmatic orifices, superior outlet of the thorax, pleural suspensory system, and the lower part of the fascial sheaths of the neck.

Although many questions remain unanswered concerning the effects of trauma, we can assume that what is true of the cerebral fluid also applies to other body fluids. Dampening of pressure occurs primarily in closed cavities such as the thorax, abdomen, and joints.

Vibratory phenomena and fluid movement

VIBRATORY WAVES

Upon traumatic impact, a large part of the applied energy is transmitted by vibrations traversing the soft and osseous tissues. The impact creates vibratory influxes which are absorbed or amplified to varying degrees depending upon the density, elasticity, plasticity, distribution, and compressibility of the tissues traversed. All elastic areas permit vibratory displacement.

In a model system, Goldsmith obtained shock waves which propagated at an approximate speed of 1.5km/s from the point of impact. Strong, abrupt impact causes vibratory waves capable of producing significant lesions. Certain lesions may be located far from the point of impact, a phenomenon well known to osteopaths.

In traumatology, fractures at the base of the skull are often seen without visible local impact. This is because the foramen magnum serves as a stress concentrator for both vertical and frontal trauma. Violent impact is transmitted through the occipital condyles to the relatively fragile base of the skull (Chapon, 1978). Even in the case of lateral cranial impact, osteopaths often find that shock waves affect abdominal organs such as the liver, spleen, and kidneys.

FLUID MOVEMENT

Acceleration and deceleration set the bodily fluids (cerebrospinal fluid, lymph, blood, etc.) in motion. Excessive pressure in the cerebrospinal fluid due to cranial deformation, in combination with sidebending movement, can cause severe lesions in the cerebral tissues. Ninety percent of acute stage concussions present an abnormality of perfusion in the frontotemporal region (Mnidiru, 1991) due to movement of intracerebral fluids and accompanying neurochemical phenomena.

Modes of Action of Trauma

Crucial factors in trauma are:

- location
- impact
- duration

- type of trauma:
  – direct mechanism through effect of contact
  – indirect mechanism through effect of inertia.

Location of impact

Studies confirm that location and type of impact are primary factors in determining severity of trauma, more so than intensity of impact. Take the example of a glass which does not break after falling from a height of one meter, yet does break after falling from a much lower spot. Although the intensity of impact is greater in the first case, the point of impact is more vulnerable in the second. The concept of location of impact is particularly important for the skull, which has specific areas of resistance and weakness.

Different types of impact

Lateral impact is most serious in the skull, because the relatively greater lateral mobility of the cervical spine increases acceleration forces. Our clinical experience indicates that lateral impact in the thorax and abdomen mostly affects the visceral attachments, that is, pleural and cervical ligaments in the thorax, and splenic, hepatic, and renal attachments in the abdomen. We believe that this is due to weak lateral mobility of the thoracic cage which affects both the abdominal and pelvic cavities.

Lateral impact causes whiplash lesions, diffuse injuries, and extradural and cerebral hematomas. The lesions produced depend primarily upon the vector of the linear or angular acceleration, which determines the direction of the head, as well as the quantity, duration, and rate of acceleration caused by the impact.

The longitudinal axis of the body has great capacity for compensation during impact. But when such compensation has reached its limit and not all the force of the trauma has been absorbed, severe lesions may result. Whiplash (from being rear-ended in a car or hit by a "rabbit punch") is the best example of this phenomenon: a great degree of anteroposterior movement causes considerable lengthening of all the longitudinal attachments of the skull and spinal column: falx cerebri, tentorium cerebelli, falx cerebelli, common anterior and posterior vertebral ligaments, and spinal cord dura mater.

Trauma as the result of contact

A list of all possible conditions resulting when trauma is due to direct contact would be very long. We will restrict our discussion to direct falls and bodily impact, and exclude lacerations, crushing wounds, and amputations. The latter pose significant problems and complications, and are not within our area of expertise.

Head

All impact to the head should be considered potentially serious. Direct impact to the skull may or may not be associated with skull fracture (cranial vault, cranial base) but even in the event of a fracture, *the severity of the damage caused to the brain is of greater importance than the injury to the bone itself.*

Locally, blows to the head are characterized by appearance of a hematoma at the point of impact and may cause loss of consciousness (initial or secondary) of variable duration and intensity, from simple momentary "blacking out" to a prolonged coma. Blows to the face can cause fractures of the facial bones, which are easy to diagnose because of hematomas, edema, or facial deformity.

Experienced osteopaths know that even in the absence of severe pathology, craniofacial bruises cause multiple disturbances of cranial mechanics. Many sutural impactions may be linked to this type of trauma. We have uncovered numerous cases of battered women solely by noting significant loss of cranial mobility with severe restrictions of the facial bones. In such cases, the patient often claims never to have fallen on the head or face, but responds affirmatively when asked "have you received a blow to the head or face." The notion of "trauma" can have a very different meaning for the practitioner than for the patient.

Pelvis

A fall on the buttocks is generally amusing to everyone except the victim. We have only to examine the popularity through the centuries of the "comic" stunt of pulling the chair out from under someone who is about to sit down. However, this type of trauma can have severe consequences for the victim. In addition to the effect of local contact, typically an ecchymosis or hematoma, an ascending shock wave reverberates through the adjacent body segments, and often affects the spinal column and base of the skull. We have found compressions between the occiput and atlas resulting from this type of trauma.

Even if the sacrum or coccyx is not fractured, the sacrococcygeal articulation may be severely affected by this type of trauma. We have lost track of the number of patients who report that their health has never been the same since experiencing a fall on the buttocks. Many symptoms can be triggered by sacrococcygeal fixation, and only a good diagnosis and clinical experience enable us to properly evaluate it in all its complexity. This type of trauma can also produce restrictions of the sacroiliac joints, changing the usual axes of mobility.

The viscera are not spared the effect of falls on the buttocks. Prolapse of the kidney is often caused or worsened by this type of impact. We once treated a patient who required a hysterectomy following such a fall. A gynecologist who had treated the patient previously was able to establish that her pain symptomatology was directly related to a trauma-induced uterine retroversion!

Trunk

Falls on the back or the upper surface of the trunk often create quite a spectacle, for they generally occur from an elevated spot such as a ladder or staircase. The impact often causes temporary respiratory incapacity such as acute dyspnea ("I had the wind knocked out of me.") The diaphragm is very sensitive to abrupt variations in pressure and therefore easily affected by such impact. Car accidents and violent games such as football often lead to traumatic impact to the trunk.

We will consider four topographical areas affected by trauma to the trunk:

- thorax
- abdomen
- pelvis
- spine

THORAX

Closed traumas of the thorax range from simple bruising to multiple rib fractures.

The severity of such lesions depends on their effect on respiratory and circulatory function.

We can distinguish:

- external lesions which affect the thoracic wall and respiratory mechanism, for example, simple or multiple rib fractures, "flail chest"
- internal lesions which affect the lungs, trachea, major vessels, or heart. Examples are pulmonary contusions, rupture of the bronchus, pleural lesions with hemothorax or pneumothorax, and cardiac contusion with tearing or displacement of the large vessels.

Respiratory problems, ranging from simple difficulty in breathing to major distress and cardiovascular difficulties such as massive internal hemorrhage, can greatly influence the prognosis.

ABDOMEN

The muscular abdominal wall transmits essentially all traumatic energy to the intraabdominal viscera. Closed abdominal trauma consist of contusions or lesions whose severity is linked to the intensity and location of the initial impact.

The nature of the lesions varies:

- in the "solid" organs (liver, spleen, and kidney): contusions and wounds, even ruptures, can cause serious internal hemorrhage
- in the "hollow" organs (stomach, intestine): ruptures, bursting, lesions of the mesenteries and mesocolons and vessels may, in addition to hemorrhage, cause infectious complications such as peritonitis.

In all cases, internal hemorrhage represents the most immediate serious risk.

PELVIS

These are closed traumas involving contusions and/or osteoarticular lesions. As in the abdomen, there is a risk of localized visceral rupture (in this case the kidney, ureter, or bladder). There is also a serious hemorrhagic risk from not only visceral lesions, but also osseous lesions, which can bleed profusely and lead to perforation of branches of the arteries.

With fractures of the iliac bones, hemorrhage from the bony region can result in a voluminous hematoma. We have witnessed the accumulation of many liters of blood, which proved life-threatening, due to a single fracture of these bones!

SPINE

Lesions of the spinal column may be isolated or associated with other lesions. They are almost always osseous or osteoarticular lesions (vertebral fracture, sprain, or subluxation) whose severity depends on neurological lesions of the cord from compression or injury by an osseous fragment.

- *High spinal lesions*, which involve the cervical spine, are likely to cause immediate or secondary cord injuries of varying severity (paraplegia, quadriplegia).

- *Low spinal lesions* of the thoracic or lumbar spine can cause paraplegia of varying severity, depending upon the level of cord injury. Osteopaths should be very familiar with the initial signs of paresthesia, tingling, and decrease in segmental muscle strength in order to avoid aggravating such lesions.

All spinal cord lesions carry a risk of sequelae, for example, paralysis.

Lower limbs

There are three major types of traumatic impact to the lower limbs:

- falls on the foot, with the lower leg extended
- falls on the knee
- impact and twisting of the leg when it is supported.

A common result in the first two cases is fracture of one or several bone segments. The bones of the lower leg are very resistant to compression, but this resistance does have a limit. The calcaneus, tibial plateau, and femoral neck are sensitive to this type of trauma, in which the concentration of stresses can exceed the bone's threshold of resistance. In a fall or impact on the knee, the knee cap is often fractured, but sometimes it is the condyle which breaks, as in "dashboard syndrome."

In the third case, ligamentous injury is more common. Sometimes this is combined with tearing of the bone. When the impact has no articular "escape mechanism," a bone shaft may fracture. The braces or taping used in some sports may cause the shaft of the femur to fracture under certain conditions.

Upper limbs

Traumatic impact affecting the upper limbs most often involves the "parachute" reaction during a forward fall. The victim lands on the hands, with wrists hyperextended. Another common scenario is a fall on the shoulder during sports or bicycle accidents. Direct impact on an upper limb may result in fracture at the point of impact. The bones here are not very resistant to compression stress.

The aftershock is propagated proximally and affects the shoulder, scapulothoracic junction, and even the thorax and cervical spine, which can focus the force of the impact on the thoracic outlet.

This area is richly supplied by the circulatory and autonomic nervous systems. Irritations following trauma to the upper limbs can promote the development of algodystrophic sequelae (combination of pain and muscle degeneration due to defective nutrition). Initially, simple traumas to the upper limbs may lead to a shoulder-hand syndrome for this reason. Interestingly, this tendency to reflex algodystrophy is less common in the lower limbs, even when trauma is more severe.

Trauma from effect of inertia 1: whiplash injury

History of a phenomenon

During recent decades, the frequency of injuries caused by sudden acceleration and deceleration has increased considerably. This is the direct result of intensive use of various methods of rapid transportation, and increasingly hectic lifestyles.

As noted in Harakal (1975), Crowe used the term *whiplash* in 1928 to describe this phenomenon in an article on injuries to the cervical spine, presented at an orthopedic conference. Macnab, the authority on this topic, defined whiplash as "primarily a deformation in extension of the cervical spine produced by sudden acceleration." He also proposed the term *acceleration extension injury,* which means "injury caused by acceleration while extended."

This type of injury is not limited to rear-end collisions in a car. With a "rabbit punch" (i.e., short chopping blow to the back of the neck or base of the skull), whiplash results from the intensive and rapid movement of the head after impact and the resulting forces of collision.

Whiplash was the focus of military studies just after World War II, in relation to catapults for ship-based airplanes. The pilots suffered temporary loss of consciousness, with sometimes disastrous results. These symptoms disappeared with the installation of headrests in airplanes.

History of a word

The word "whiplash" evokes images of the "lash of a whip." It designates a traumatic series of events in which the cephalic part of the body, which is free, is suddenly mobilized relative to the caudad part, which is relatively fixed or less free.

In this type of complex mechanical system, an accumulation of kinetic energy is added to the most mobile segments, set in motion by inertia. The focus of energy on the final mobile part of the system is illustrated by the lashing of a whip. Simple propagation of a small impulse from the handle toward the free end of the lash produces a snap from the arrival of the shock wave. The shock wave at the free end is due to acceleration.

While this term is widely used in the allopathic world, a wide gulf has developed between the common usage of this term in European osteopathy and in the conventional medical world. At one extreme, for a number of our osteopathic colleagues, "everything is whiplash." At the other, for orthopedists and traumatologists, whiplash is the exclusive domain of skull trauma and the term is used only in regard to patients with severe post-concussion syndromes.

The meaning of this term is constantly evolving, as reflected in the published studies on the subject. We need to be clear about our usage of the term.

Lesion mechanism of whiplash injury

TRADITIONAL CONCEPT

In English, the term "whiplash" traditionally refers to a shock wave triggered by trauma, and its consequences. Whiplash requires acceleration, that is, sudden variation in speed. The two common scenarios are:

- a moving body is suddenly stopped
- a body at rest is suddenly put into motion.

These phenomena occur daily during automobile rides. The great diversity in impact, trajectory, and acceleration makes it impossible for us to discuss all the possible manifestations.

In the traditional osteopathic approach to whiplash, according to Heilig (1963), there are two phases *(Fig. 1-11).* Consider the example of a rear-end vehicular collision:

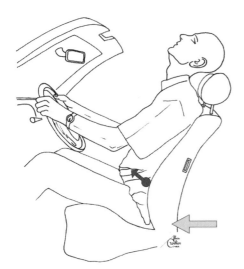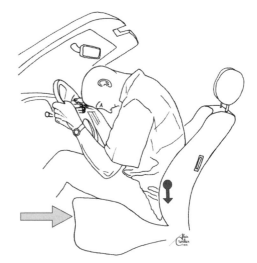

Snapping back: the center of gravity
is projected upward and forward.

Whipping forward: the center of gravity
suddenly descends toward the ground.

Fig. 1-11: The two basic types of whiplash

Phase 1: sudden acceleration of the lower half of the body toward the front with resulting posterior movement of the head ("snapping back"), until it recovers its initial acceleration, slowed down by its own inertia.

Phase 2: anterior movement ("whipping forward") of the head immediately after deceleration of the lower part of the body. The whiplash phenomenon is more intense if the deceleration is sudden, or if an obstacle is hit head on.

In this approach, whiplash can involve any combination of the following:

- sudden acceleration of the lower half of the body
- resistance of upper parts of the body through inertia
- deformation in one direction
- change in the direction of acceleration
- change in the direction of deformation.

We believe that the term whiplash should be reserved for this type of phenomenon. Some other term should be used to designate the general effects of trauma on the body or specific tissues.

DIFFERENT TYPES OF WHIPLASH

Depending upon the direction of applied forces, four types of whiplash can be theoretically distinguished:

- posteroanterior (back to front) whiplash
- anteroposterior (front to back) whiplash
- lateral whiplash from right to left
- lateral whiplash from left to right.

In clinical practice, none of these four types occurs in isolation.

MODERN CONCEPT

Whiplash has often been thought to result from a shock wave which traverses the body as the result of direct trauma. In our opinion, the original definition refers only to traumatic mechanisms in which the phenomenon of inertia predominates, and causes tissue lesions subsequent to acceleration and deceleration. The term "whiplash" should not be applied to direct bodily collisions in which phenomena of contact are of major significance, as in a fall on the buttocks or the back.

A more modern definition of whiplash was given by our late colleague Lionnelle Issartel. She defined it as involving "sudden acceleration or deceleration applied to the human body which is not prepared for such an event." In this sense, whiplash is defined by rapid and unexpected passage from a state of rest to a state of movement, and vice versa.

The notion of "lack of preparedness" is of primary importance in whiplash. Because the neuromuscular circuits are not ready to confront the impact mechanism, the inertia of the body segments controls the various consequent deformations. Whiplash can also occur when the magnitude of the trauma surpasses the protective capacity of the neuromuscular system, even when the person anticipates the impact.

By extension, whiplash can refer to a sudden change in movement involving the entire body. The osteopathic approach to trauma and illness is based upon the concept of a physiologic-anatomic relationship governing homeostasis and bodily function. We should view whiplash as a lesion affecting the whole body, resulting from the introduction of energy into the system. It may disrupt equilibrium of all physiologic and anatomic homeostatic mechanisms.

PATHOPHYSIOLOGY AND THE DEVELOPMENT OF RESTRICTIONS

If acceleration of the lower part of the body is very rapid, the anterior structures will be most greatly deformed. From the effect of traction, tissue microtears can occur in the anterior anatomic structures, while posteriorly, the osseous elements are affected primarily by compression. During the second phase, with sudden deceleration, the stresses of traction and microtears affect the posterior structures, while compression affects anterior structures such as the intervertebral disks and vertebral bodies.

As noted by Wright (1956), studies carried out by the U.S. Air Force demonstrated that resistance capacity to acceleration in flexion is approximately 50 g, whereas resistance capacity to acceleration in extension is only 5 g—ten times less. This explains why most lesions occur during backward movement of the head, as observed in our clinical practice.

The position of the subject at the moment of impact is also crucial; it determines lateral, asymmetric (left or right dominating), or bilaterally symmetric deformations. A simple variation in head position will determine which side of the neck is affected by whiplash. Likewise, the position of the upper limbs plays a major role in thoracic or costal lesions or injuries of the pectoral girdle.

Experiments by the U.S. Air Force demonstrated that it is possible to apply deceleration until 35 g without causing injury, sometimes even up to 75 g! In the great majority of automobile accidents, the forces of deceleration are 25 g or less, that is, within limits tolerable by the human body, but *only when the body is suitably braced and supported.*

Presence or absence of a headrest plays a key role in whiplash injuries. Head support limits posterior whiplash injury and decreases trauma during the first phase. Without head support, tolerance to impact is much less. In certain situations the seat belt can cause the forces of whiplash to converge on the pectoral girdle and superior thoracic outlet.

Clinical practice

As mentioned above, the term "whiplash" has been used with many different meanings, and a certain amount of confusion naturally exists. It is important to be aware of the difference in English usage between the term *whiplash*, which designates the mechanism of lesion, and *whiplash injury*, which indicates the injuries resulting from whiplash. Hearing some practitioners of manual medicine say that their patient has "whiplash" is about as informative as hearing that someone was "hit over the head" or "fell on their rear end."

As noted above, we prefer to use the term "whiplash" to designate a whole-body mechanism which may involve a series of related vertebral, paravertebral, craniosacral, vascular, and visceral restrictions. It does not refer to a typical syndrome nor a specific injury. One defining characteristic is as a *phenomenon of inertia which predominates to the exclusion of contact phenomena.*

The damage caused by whiplash ranges from simple muscle stretching to bone fracture, and includes rupture of ligaments or blood vessels. Severe cases can result in quadriplegia, coma, or even death by decerebration.

The more rapid the whiplash, the more pathogenic. With very rapid whiplash the victim may feel a sensation of tearing, internal sprain, or even intracavity or interosseous explosion or implosion. This last sensation is usually accompanied by a feeling of emptiness or absence.

The great variety in degrees of whiplash injury causes forensic problems. There is often no manifest lesion that can be objectively documented. The minor changes seen on x-ray may not account for the symptoms reported by the patient. We have heard from many patients of their great distress at being unable to find a sympathetic ear to listen to their symptoms, their need to seek repeated medical assessments and second opinions, and their difficulty in obtaining reimbursement from insurance companies for injuries.

These problems underscore the importance of the osteopathic approach. Examination for loss of mobility, limitation of movement, level of injury, and depth of restriction constitutes a major part of the diagnosis. These are documentable dysfunctions that not only facilitate effective treatment, but also objectify the patients' complaints, which is psychologically important.

Etiology

Whiplash injury does not occur automatically following a fall or collision. It occurs following a sudden change (rapid acceleration or deceleration) which involves the entire person. As mentioned above, an essential point is that the victim is not prepared for this sudden change, and protective neurosensory and motor circuits are not "on alert" when the event occurs.

Some common causes of whiplash injury are cited by H. Magoun (1976) and L. Issartel (1983):

- automobile accidents
- missing a step in the dark, with unexpected downward acceleration
- being caught in a rip tide while swimming, and thrown around by the surf
- jumping improperly on a trampoline, with body extension exceeding its physiological limits
- amusement park rides which combine acceleration, braking, moment of inertia, and centrifugal force, with potential damage to young anatomic structures. Even though the neurological circuits are alert, a lack of effective visual reference points in this type of ride facilitates whiplash.
- encountering a major air pocket or violent turbulence as an airplane passenger. We recall a news story of an airplane which had to make an emergency landing to unload passengers seriously injured as a result of major turbulence. Skull trauma and cervical sprains were diagnosed in several passengers who had not fastened their seat belts.
- diving into deep water, with a sudden change in direction immediately after entering the water, or impact of the head against the bottom
- vigorously slapping the buttocks of a newborn while holding him by the feet in an attempt to stimulate respiration.

These situations do not necessarily cause a whiplash injury! The human body and tissues have excellent compensation/adaptation mechanisms. Whiplash is less likely if the disturbance is not very violent, is not repetitive, and if the person has activated his neuromuscular circuits in anticipation of impact.

Certain factors and symptoms during traumatic events contribute to or are associated with *damaging whiplash injury:*

- longer duration of impact or collision. Inertia can be more damaging than force of the impact.
- post-traumatic dyspnea or having one's "wind knocked out"
- loss of consciousness (even brief), sensation of malaise, or profound dizziness
- perception of a "flint stone" or "burnt" smell immediately after trauma. This reflects damage to the olfactory nerves during the shock and aftershock.
- post-traumatic nausea and vomiting
- post-traumatic episodes of confusion
- sensorimotor signs such as tingling, paresthesia, or paresis, even without objective evidence at the neurological examination, during the hours or days following the accident.

The more of these signs of whiplash injury that are present, the greater the likelihood of pathological effects or post-traumatic syndromes.

Symptomatology

H. Magoun (1976) distinguishes between severe and benign whiplash injury. The latter type affects mainly the soft tissues, and includes sprains and stretching. In benign whiplash cases, the victim may undergo a moderately severe collision but present no signs immediately after the accident. During the first few hours the symptomatology is unremarkable, aside from possible nervous reactions. After several hours, the victim reports soreness, with fatigue, or stiffness sometimes accompanied by nausea. In subsequent days, if sufficient edema has developed, the stiffness causes a loss of mobility in the cervical spine, with pain upon simple pressure on the muscle mass. Suboccipital headaches accompany the muscle spasms and irritations of upper cervical nerves.

More severe injuries involve the intervertebral disks, interapophyseal joints and ligaments. Symptoms are of more rapid onset. Pain, stiffness, torticollis, radicular pain, segmental neuralgias (particularly in the suboccipital region), nausea, vomiting, headaches, and psychological manifestations may be present. Pain may radiate anywhere, depending upon the tissue damaged. Numbness or paresthesias of the arms and legs may appear, and, more rarely, muscular paresis or even paraplegia.

The patient keeps her head rigid. Cephalic symptoms may include dizziness, ringing or buzzing in the ears, visual disturbances, lightheadedness, hearing loss, shooting pains in the upper cranium, and signs of neurological damage. It is not uncommon to note difficulties with concentration, confusion, disorientation, or even loss of consciousness.

Because of the degenerative phenomena to which they are subject, older persons are frequently more incapacitated than young persons by the same degree of trauma. They may present symptoms which appear months or years after the accident.

Diagnosis of whiplash injury

Based upon the history, reported symptoms, and various motion tests at our disposal, we attempt to reach a diagnosis. We use a qualitative score system for evaluation, with four possible conclusions:

- whiplash injury excluded
- whiplash injury possible
- whiplash injury probable
- whiplash injury certain.

Effects of whiplash on the primary respiratory mechanism (PRM)

Mechanical disorders can be demonstrated in the spinal axis and the thorax during vertebral articular diagnosis. However, as Magoun (1976) notes:

> No neck injury will return to normal if the occiput above and the spine and the sacrum below remain uncorrected. Body metabolism will not resume proper function if the fascia remains restricted and the internal respiration continues to be stagnated. All of this must be very gently done.

If we envision treatment of the sequelae of whiplash only in terms of vertebral manipulation, we see only a part of the pathology, and we cannot expect to achieve lasting results.

Following whiplash, we frequently note significant tension of the spinal cord dura mater. This tension affects the vertebral mechanism directly, and may thereby affect the craniosacral mechanism.

The PRM is commonly affected by anteroposterior whiplash (e.g., from a rear-end collision), which can be divided into two phases.

- During the first phase, as a result of the impact and acceleration, the skull, spinal column, and sacrum are drawn upwards, decreasing the effective weight of the body segments involved (Fig. 1-12a).

- During the second phase, deceleration and gravity put the skull and spine into flexion, restoring the real weight of the body segments *(Fig. 1-12b)*.

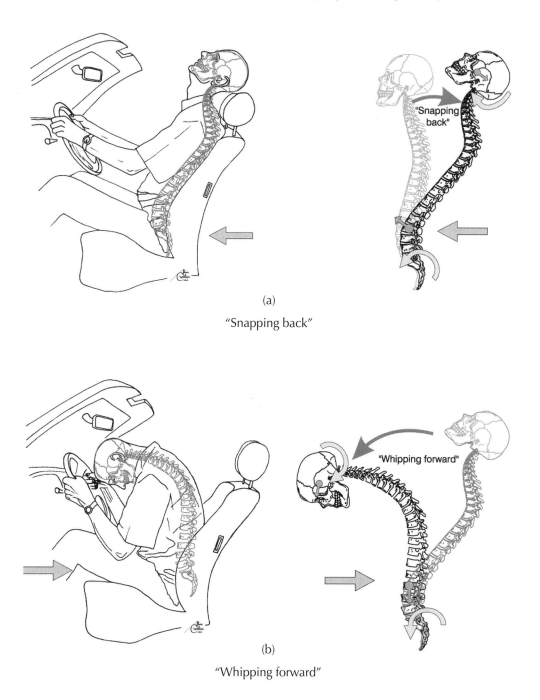

(a)

"Snapping back"

(b)

"Whipping forward"

Fig. 1-12: Whiplash: two types of productive mechanism

First phase

- The spinal complex is extended globally.
- At the sacroiliac level, due to an increase in lordosis, the sacral base plunges anteriorly following a mechanical flexion movement. This movement of the sacrum between the iliac bones corresponds to extension of the PRM.
- On the occipitoatloid level, mechanical extension of the cervical spine pushes the lower part of the occipital squama anteriorly, which corresponds to flexion of the PRM.

Second phase

- Because of deceleration and the weight of the trunk, the sacrum tends to become embedded between the ilia, fixing the PRM position of extension acquired during the first phase.
- At the cervical/cephalic level, sudden deceleration causes the head to "fall down" on C1. The occiput, which is in a position of PRM flexion, is embedded between the temporals. The petrobasilar and petrojugular sutures are compressed, which affects the content of the foramen lacerum posterius. Severe cases may involve compression of the sphenobasilar symphysis or an inferior vertical strain.

The antagonistic positions of the occiput and the sacrum complicate the cycles of flexion (expansion) and extension (relaxation) of the craniosacral mechanism, and create an overload of constraining tension on the dura mater of the spinal cord. Alteration of cranial venous drainage, cranial nerve activity, and tension of the spinal column may unbalance the vertebral mechanism. All these disturbances break the harmony of the PRM and impair the body's internal self-regulating capacity.

REFLECTIONS ON WHIPLASH AND THE PRM

It is important to recognize whiplash injury as a true clinical entity. To some practitioners, asynchrony in the craniosacral system is seen as the *only factor* confirming whiplash. We consider this as just one symptom among many. The cause of the asynchrony needs to be diagnosed to restore PRM physiology. Certain vertebral restrictions, such as translational or bilateral ones (known as Type III lesions in Europe), induce tension of the spinal cord dura mater and disturb the PRM. The perception of craniosacral asynchrony is therefore not diagnostic of a whiplash injury.

We view whiplash injury as a superposition of articular, neuromuscular, fascial, and fluid disorders which interconnect like a series of Russian dolls one inside the next. It is difficult to appreciate the number of levels involved, and essentially impossible to "release the whiplash" during an initial treatment session—or even after a single manipulation, as some osteopaths claim! Restoration of craniosacral harmony should be considered as the ultimate goal of treatment, not as a simple therapeutic stage.

It is perhaps preferable to reserve the term "whiplash injury" for serious cases and to use a different term designating less severe, post-traumatic sequelae. Referring to all cases as whiplash injury causes this term to lose its significance.

We are not convinced of the physical and mechanical reality of the concept of craniosacral asynchrony. The dura mater is not very extendible, and it seems unlikely that it can have a degree of inertia to the extent of not simultaneously transmitting the PRM to the two poles of the spinal cord.

Another hypothesis can be suggested regarding the motility of the central nervous system. During craniosacral listening, we feel the kinetic expression of the brain's motility with the occipital hand. But what does the sacral hand feel? Merely transmission of the cranial PRM to the sacrum via the spinal cord dura mater? Perhaps we also feel the expression of the motility of the spinal cord, roots, nerves, etc. After certain cases of whiplash, it seems likely that motility of these two segments of the central nervous system can lose their synchrony. We would then feel a system which is not communicating on the level of tissue motility, and our hands would register a displacement between the sacrum and occiput.

It is often difficult to convey a sensation verbally, and we must beware of cliches. However, our experience is that contradictory physiological situations of the sacrum and occiput can lead to a sensation that one or both of these structures is "frozen," hypomobile, or dense. This produces disturbance of PRM perception, even more so if the spinal cord dura mater is significantly tense.

Trauma from effect of inertia 2: "blast injury" and barotrauma

This type of trauma results from sudden application of pressure to the body. Injury rates for miners and professional users of explosives have declined in recent decades, but there are still many people injured by explosives in industrial accidents or terrorist attacks.

In this case, the shock wave is caused by the explosion from the blast, which sometimes throws victims far from their original location. The pressure affects the entire body and damage to the tissues is considerable. Acceleration can be significant and similar to whiplash. A variety of injuries such as fractures, wounds, and amputation may occur.

Naturally, the ear is particularly vulnerable to barotrauma. The tympanic membrane can be easily perforated by excessive pressure. Damage to the middle and inner ear leads to acoustic as well as vestibular dysfunction.

Other types of trauma

Pregnancy-related and obstetrical causes

OBSTETRICAL STRAINS

Unfortunately, birth can still be one of the most traumatic of life's experiences. We have written many times of the disastrous effects of forceps deliveries or other forceful maneuvers designed to expel or disengage the fetus. This type of entry into the world can have long-lasting physical and psychological effects on the child. We believe there are real correlations between such neonatal trauma and pathologies which we treat much later in life.

INTRAUTERINE STRAINS

Trauma is often related to pregnancy. Forceful trauma, fear, or terror experienced by the mother can be transmitted to the baby. Furthermore, although some deny it, contractions prior to the actual birthing period are not physiological and are sometimes catastrophic for the mechanical equilibrium of the fetus. According to our American colleague Viola Frymann (1996), these contractions typically produce compressions of the sacrum, base of the skull, or both. The configuration of the mother's pelvis, or presence of a uterine fibroid, can also create compressions which are damaging to the fetus.

Prematurity can constitute an aggravating factor. Certain obstetrical manipulations which are well tolerated by a full-term infant may be mechanically damaging to a fetus which is even two weeks premature. Duration of labor and rapidity of the birth process are also important factors. A short labor and quick delivery mean less potential trauma for the baby.

EMOTIONS AND FEAR

In our high-stress society, many people undergo significant psychological trauma at some point in their lives. Being a victim or witness of a major accident, assault, homicide, or other violent episode sometimes engenders intense reactions which are manifested physically as well as psychologically.

Although this type of trauma does not fall within the scope of this book, we want to emphasize the fact that any emotion can have physical consequences. While some of our colleagues have created the term "emotional whiplash" for these situations, we prefer to reserve use of the term "whiplash" for cases of physical trauma, as discussed above.

Chapter Two:
A Functional-Anatomical Approach to Trauma

Table of Contents

A Functional-Anatomical
Approach to Trauma

The Skull and Its Susceptibility to Fracture

The skull provides its priceless contents—the brain—maximal protection against impact. Its rigidity depends upon the thickness, hardness, and form of the bone. The sutures play a crucial role in absorbing and dissipating impact *(Figs. 2-1 to 2-4)*. Without them, the skull would fracture from a relatively minor blow. The skull is most elastic in its transverse diameter, which can change by as much as one centimeter.

Anatomic configuration of the skull

The great French anatomist Testut (1896) compared the skull to a boat with a keel, in that it has a strongly reinforced basilar section and more fragile slats.

Reinforced areas

- inferiorly: the basilar region extending from the foramen magnum to the sella turcica is reinforced by other attached bony masses
- anteriorly: the frontoethmoidal region, excluding the cribriform plate
- posteriorly: the occipital region, excluding the posterior section of each condyle
- anterolaterally: the orbitosphenoidal region (protected by the sphenoid wings)
- posterolaterally: the petromastoid region (excluding the petrous bone area hollowed out by the ear cavity).

More fragile areas

These are the "slats" from Testut's analogy, and consist of the following regions:

- sphenofrontal
- petrosphenoid
- petrooccipital.

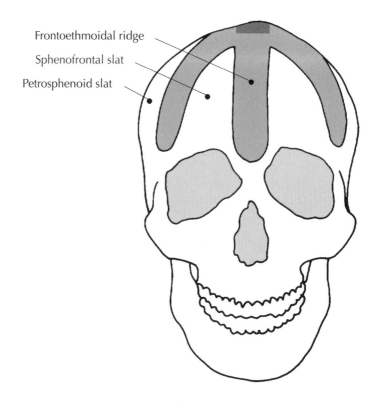

Frontoethmoidal ridge
Sphenofrontal slat
Petrosphenoid slat

Fig. 2-1: Anterior view of skull

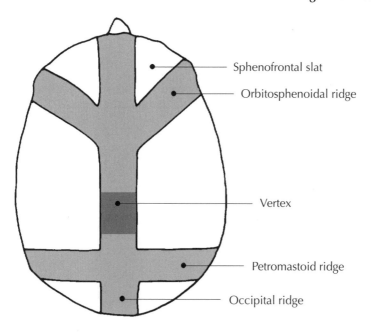

Sphenofrontal slat
Orbitosphenoidal ridge

Vertex

Petromastoid ridge

Occipital ridge

Fig. 2-2: Superior view of skull

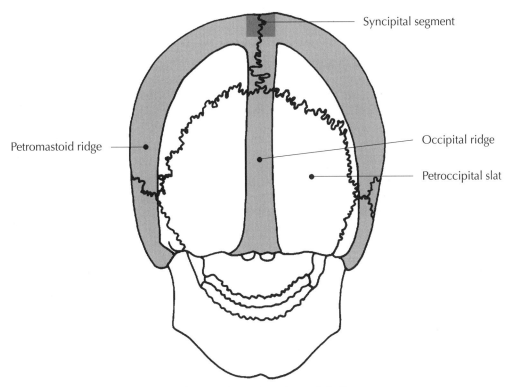

Fig. 2-3: Posterior view of skull

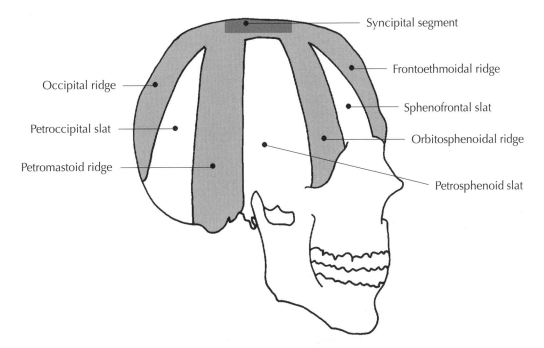

Fig. 2-4: Lateral view of skull

In Testut's time cranial trauma related to transportation had less serious consequences than it has today, since vehicles of that time were much slower. Today, cranial lesions most commonly occur at the frontal, temporoapical, and temporobasal regions, the junction of the falx in the cingulate gyrus, the inferomedial surface of the temporal lobe, and the junction of the tentorium with the apex of the petrous portion of the temporal bone. While the thinner sections are more deformable and more likely to fracture, trauma to these areas is less likely to generate significant shock waves than trauma to the reinforced areas.

Mechanism of skull fracture

During impact, the dimensions of the skull decrease along the axis of impact and increase in the perpendicular direction. The flat bones of the skull contain inner and outer layers of compact bone tissue, known as the inner and outer tables respectively. During fracture, the inner table is the first to break, followed by the outer table. Testut used the analogy of a flexible branch which bends before breaking. As with a branch, it is the section located in the concavity that is the first to break. That is, the inner table fractures more easily since its arc of bending is more acute than that of the outer table. This detail demonstrates the involvement of the dura mater in the mechanism of fracture, a fact that may not appear significant in nonosteopathic diagnostic approaches. Because the dura mater attaches to the internal surface of the bone, whenever the bone bends in response to trauma, the dura bends with a more acute arc. This means that it can, with relative ease, separate from the bony surface or tear longitudinally.

Severity of fractures

One might assume that, during trauma, a more fragile bony region will undergo greater tissue damage than a more solid section, but this is not always the case. *Note:* The severity of injury from a fracture is due not to the fracture itself but rather to the associated neuronal, vascular, or dura mater damage.

A fracture results from the initiation, concentration, and sudden release of energy. In certain cases the prognosis for cranial trauma is better if a fracture has occurred, in that the force of the trauma has been released in the fracturing process. In cranial trauma without fracture the forces exerted remain captive; that is, since they are not released in a fracture, they wreak more havoc in the intracranial soft tissues. We will discuss this phenomenon in more detail in Chapter 3 below.

Intracranial hematomas caused by fractures are a major concern in emergency situations. Hematomas can be:

- extradural (between the bone and dura mater)
- subdural (under the dura mater)
- intracerebral (in the cerebral tissue itself).

Container-Content Relationship of the Skull

The skull and its contents have different degrees of inertia because of their different densities.

Like water, the intracranial contents are not easily compressible. The brain is a viscoelastic tissue. Deformation of the cranial cavity causes movement of the cerebral mass and the cerebrospinal fluid, especially toward the largest opening—the foramen magnum—which provides a kind of "escape valve." We believe that, depending upon the direction of impact and propagation of the shock wave, other cranial openings may compensate for excessive pressure and intracranial cerebral mobilization. For example, even though compensation and mobilization are stronger in the foramen magnum, they also occur in the ocular and auditory orifices.

Internal surface of the skull

This surface is not smooth or uniform. During movement, the cerebral mass will press against irregularities and osseous obstacles. The major risk of lesion occurs at the surface of the anterior and middle fossae, where sensory receptors may be destroyed by movement of the cerebral mass.

Cerebrospinal fluid (CSF)

The CSF can be considered the third liquid environment of the body. Like the blood and lymph, it has important mechanical functions; for example, it enables the intracranial segments to coexist in harmony with the osseous walls. Depending on the person, the brain contains 90-150g of CSF (slightly more in older people), and CSF production is between 500-850ml per day. This means that CSF is replaced 4-5 times per day.

CSF volume and pressure

The skull is a rigid structure of fixed volume, containing three components:

- cerebral tissue (volume 1400cm^3 on average)
- intracranial vascular volume (75cm^3)
- CSF (75cm^3)

Intracranial vascular and CSF volume may vary without causing serious problems. In fact, our observations lead us to believe that these two volumes vary inversely to maintain acceptable intracranial pressure, as stated in the Monro-Kellie hypothesis (Livingston, 1965; Schuller, 1993).

Average cranial CSF pressure must always be higher than atmospheric pressure to avoid compression of the cerebral mass. It is 150mm H_2O in normal standing, somewhat higher in the seated position, and may reach 200mm H_2O in unusual situations.

CSF pressure is generally measured at the lumbar level, with the subject in horizontal (lateral decubitus) position. Its average value in this position in an adult is 150mm H_2O; values between 60-180mm H_2O are considered normal by most authors.

In seated position, the average is 300mm H_2O in an adult, between 40 to 80mm in a child under six, and between 15 to 80mm in a newborn. Pressure is lower in the large cistern (119mm average; range 41-197mm), and in the ventricles (50-180mm). Pressure is greatly influenced by patient position:

- in prone position, pressure is decreased (by 80mm H_2O) relative to that noted in lateral decubitus position
- in supine position, pressure is increased by a similar amount.

Bradley demonstrated that CSF pressure in the coronal suture is 30mm H_2O in a patient in supine position. Flexion-elevation of the head lowers the pressure to -60mm

H_2O and extension increases it to +120mm H_2O. Similar effects are obtained on a tilting table. In fact, any variation in weight modifies CSF pressure, which is important for understanding mechanisms of trauma. Cats subjected to centrifugal forces of -6 g to +6 g demonstrate variations in pressure from +80 to -190mm H_2O relative to normal. Such variation helps explain the immediate effects of whiplash trauma, which can cause intracranial pressure to vary rapidly (Schuller, 1993).

CSF secretion and resorption

Secretion is independent of CSF pressure, but resorption is directly proportional to it. Resorption ceases below 68mm H_2O, which corresponds to intracranial venous sinus pressure.

Sixty percent of any increase in pressure caused by occlusion of the jugular veins is transmitted to the CSF. Any variation in intrathoracic pressure immediately affects CSF pressure, since the nonvalvular venous network is drained by the superior vena cava. This occurs during physiological events such as coughing, and significant muscular efforts such as defecation.

Functions of CSF

Protection and maintenance

CSF has an important protective function. All the elements of the central and peripheral nervous system are bathed in CSF, which protects them against mechanical and traumatic assault. The brain is literally "in suspension" in the CSF. It has been determined that the weight of an isolated brain in air is 1.5kg. Supported by the CSF, its effective weight is *no more than 50g!* How can we fail to be astonished by such a phenomenon!

The spinal cord weighs only 30-40g. The CSF does not significantly affect its weight, but does protect it against mechanical assault. In fact, spinal compartment CSF volume is ~80ml per 25ml of cord, while cerebral compartment CSF volume is only ~60ml per 1500ml of encephalon.

Dampening of pressure

Although some pressure gradients compensated for by the CSF are due to trauma, most are caused by differences in vascular pressure. The CSF supplies negative intra-thoracic pressure and a turgor effect for the abdominal organs. Concepts relating to Archimedean buoyant force caused by the CSF are discussed in the section on neuro-meningeal dynamics below.

Protection during cranial trauma

The CSF protects the brain and spinal cord from direct and indirect impact. As mentioned above, during direct impact, the skull is deformed by compression in the direction of impact and widening in the perpendicular direction. The CSF is pushed primarily toward the subarachnoid cisternae at the base of the brain ("basal cisternae"). CSF circulates around the brain in various sulci, rivulets, banks, and flows which are directed toward six cisternae: the supracallosal cistern, cistern of the lamina terminalis, cistern of the great cerebral vein, interpeduncular cistern, pontine cistern, and cerebello-medullary cistern. All these cisternae communicate with one another and with the fourth ventricle, which is a frequent focus of osteopathic treatment.

During trauma, the CSF is primarily pushed backward. The fourth ventricle suddenly receives most of the CSF from the lateral ventricles. When the impact is violent, distention of the fourth ventricle causes inhibition of cerebral and bulbar function, with results ranging from simple syncope to potentially fatal cardiorespiratory arrest. If cardiorespiratory functions are affected, a cerebral concussion may occur. Forceful impact of the CSF on certain sections of the brain seems to cause release of catecholamines and endorphins.

Nutritional, immunological, and hormonal functions

The CSF nourishes the arachnoid and ependymal cells of the pia mater, and controls the chemical environment of the central nervous system (CNS) by eliminating wastes. During its circulation, CSF undergoes changes of pH and electrolyte composition. It is sensitive to carbon dioxide levels and venous pressure. CSF may also provide immunological (cellular and humoral) protection for the CNS, in analogy to the lymphatic system of the body.

Numerous substances are excreted into the CNS, as they are into the body's circulatory system. The concept of the CSF as a "sink" is actually quite old. CSF is replaced 4-5 times per day, as mentioned above, and thereby helps control the chemical composition of different regions of the CNS and contributes to "cleaning" of the brain.

CSF also plays an important role as a neuroendocrine carrier. This path is used by most of the "releasing factors," and perhaps also by the sleep mediators. It is less well known that the CSF plays a role as a regulator for the hormones and endorphins secreted by the hypothalamus, pituitary gland, and pineal gland. It is quite likely that the many neurotransmitters identified in the CSF use it for their transport.

CSF pulsations

Osteopaths sometimes seem to think that we are the only professionals interested in movements of the CSF. Of course, this is not the case. One very important researcher in this field who is not associated with osteopathy is Professor Claude Manelfe of the Central University Hospital in Toulouse. His work is described below.

Oscillatory or pulsatile movements of CSF at the level of the spinal cord were known even before the development of magnetic resonance imaging (MRI). They were attributed to systolic ejection of CSF from the third ventricle, influenced by thalamic pulsations from arterial waves reaching the brain. More recently, it was demonstrated that CSF drainage from the lateral ventricles toward the third ventricle, cerebral aqueduct, fourth ventricle, and basal cisternae derives from a cyclical forward and backward movement with each heartbeat (caudad during systole, cephalad during diastole).

The volume of fluid leaving the ventricles with each heartbeat is equal to the amount of CSF produced at the ventricular level. The pulsatile movement may be due to the action of the brain itself on the lateral ventricles, *caused by its motility*. The pulsations at the level of the cervical and thoracic spine are caused by pulsatile movement of the brainstem in the basal cisternae.

Manelfe's experiments

Using MRI, Manelfe demonstrated the existence of a descending systolic wave (100 to 300msec following the R wave of the electrocardiogram), with a maximum speed of ~1.5cm/s at the level of the interpeduncular cistern. The latter is followed, after a brief period of CSF immobility (400 to 500msec after the R wave) by an ascending wave (600msec until the end of the diastole). These pulsations propagate freely in the spinal subarachnoid space, communicating primarily with the basal cisternae (Manelfe, 1989).

Movement of the brain upon impact

Experimental and clinical data have demonstrated that during traumatic impact the brain tends to move forward and backward inside the skull. The CSF and meninges dampen, limit, and orient this movement. Specifically, the CSF dampens the effect of the impact force, and the membrane system takes over when the dampening limit has been reached. The meninges, especially the falx cerebri and tentorium cerebelli, help prevent excessive movement of the brain.

The intensity and direction of impact affect the degree of damage caused by movement of the cerebral mass. Movement or acceleration of the brain in rotation or sidebending can induce lengthening of the brain on its sagittal axis.

Because of the effects of acceleration and deceleration, anteroposterior types of impact (e.g., whiplash) which are accompanied by rotation have serious consequences throughout the spinal canal. Such cases are most likely to produce intracavity (luminal) cerebrospinal shock waves, which push against natural bony or pathological contours.

When the shock wave begins in the skull, the resulting lesions can be either cerebral or vertebral. At the vertebral level, they tend to be localized in the areas of spinal curvature change at C5-C6 and T8-T9. When the shock wave begins in the lower limbs, sacrum, coccyx, or pelvis and moves upward, it tends to be concentrated in the area of curvature change at T12-L1. These observations explain, in part, the frequency with which these vertebrae are fractured.

Role of the foramen magnum and the free border of the tentorium cerebelli

During significant impact, the medulla oblongata and middle part of the cerebellum move toward the spinal canal. This movement is provoked by displacement of the cerebral mass and consequent increase in intracranial CSF pressure, and permitted by the foramen magnum.

A moving cerebral mass has few escape mechanisms inside the skull, other than the foramen magnum. The largest part of the cerebral mass is in the posterior fossa, and the forces during impact converge toward the free border of the tentorium cerebelli (the dura mater which supports the occipital lobes and covers the cerebellum). The bulbo-cerebellar, subtentorial region is thus projected toward the foramen magnum, as seen in some cases of bulbar trauma.

When the direction of impact is complex, especially if transverse, the auditory openings help to compensate for the movement of the cerebral mass and to dampen the shock wave of collision. The ocular openings seem to be less important in this regard.

In significant trauma, the forces of collision are concentrated toward the foramen magnum, and the posterior section of the dura mater resists posterior movement of the cerebral mass. For this reason, the posterior part of the falx and the dura mater surrounding the foramen magnum need to be treated afterward.

In summary, the foramen magnum, falx cerebri, tentorium cerebelli, bony irregularities of the cranium and vertebrae, and to a lesser extent the auditory and ocular openings regulate or concentrate intracranial forces during a collision.

Functional Anatomy of the CNS

Meningeal system

The meningeal system, especially the dura mater, is, in our opinion, a key element in traumatic tissue restrictions and their treatment. We will review several points necessary to fully understand and effectively treat this region.

General organization

The meninges derive from the somatopleure, while the embryonic layer of the brainstem is derived from the splanchnopleure. The three embryonic meningeal layers—pia mater, arachnoid, and dura mater—surround the entire CNS.

Histologically speaking, the three embryonic layers are very different:

- the dura mater is a fibrous membrane
- the pia mater is a cellular-vascular membrane
- the arachnoid, which was long described as serous after the work of the famous early 20th-century French anatomist Bichat, is in fact a nonvascular connective tissue membrane.

The dura mater and arachnoid are contiguous with each other. The subarachnoid space between the arachnoid and pia mater contains CSF.

Pia mater

The pia mater is a resistant membrane composed of two layers (one longitudinal, one circular) of connective tissue fibers. It is closely adherent to the spinal cord, follows its contours, and constitutes its external limit. The pia matter carries numerous vessels.

An important component of pia mater are the *dentate ligaments*. Situated laterally, they are supported by the pia mater and adhere to its deep surface by digitations situated between the dural orifices of the nerve root exits. They anchor the spinal cord to the pia mater, thereby guaranteeing transverse centering of the spinal cord in the vertebral canal regardless of the position of the spinal column.

Arachnoid

Although long described as a serous membrane, recent studies demonstrate that it is in fact a connective tissue membrane without vessels or nerves. It is composed of two layers:

- an external layer composed of flattened endothelial cells
- an internal layer made up of interconnected connective tissue fibers in a dense network.

Like the cornea, the arachnoid depends for its nutrition on the fluid environment which surrounds it: the CSF. Its major function is to protect the CSF environment and provide one boundary for the subarachnoid space which contains the CSF. Its connective tissue fibroblast cells are capable of proliferating and containing or isolating threatening organisms or foreign bodies.

Dura mater

The dura mater is divided into cranial and spinal portions *(Fig. 2-5)*. Although these are interconnected by many fibers and have a reciprocal tension relationship, we cannot say that they are really continuous. Rather, they are like two closely linked muscles which work together. We will discuss the spinal portion first.

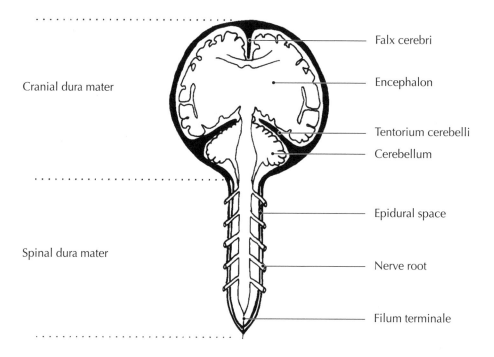

Fig. 2-5: General organization of the dura mater

SPINAL DURA MATER

This is Sutherland's "core link" (also known as the central link or deep link). It is a hollow cylinder which contains the medulla oblongata at its upper end and extends from the occiput to S2-S3, where it tapers to form a dural cul-de-sac, contained in the sacral canal. Since the spinal cord does not extend past L2, the capacity of the spinal dura mater is much greater than the volume of the medulla oblongata and the spinal cord.

The dural sheath is punctured laterally by a series of orifices corresponding to the passage of nerve roots toward the vertebral foramina. Two parts can be differentiated: the collar marking the exit orifice, and the radicular dural sheath. The latter, shorter than the root, accompanies it as far as the vertebral foramen, where it is continued by the perineurium.

DURAL SHEATH

The external surface of this sheath is composed of vascular adipose tissue: it is a semifluid structure, filling the epidural space and separating it from the walls of the vertebral canal. The epidural space contains fat and an intraspinal venous plexus. The dura mater is attached to the common posterior vertebral ligament by fibrous prolongations, which are especially numerous in the lumbar and cervical regions.

The internal surface of the sheath is covered by the parietal embryonic layer of the arachnoid.

STRUCTURE OF THE SPINAL CORD DURA MATER

This fibrous and resistant sheath has a structure which is different from its cranial homologue. According to Maillot (1990), it corresponds to the internal, purely meningeal part of the cranial dura mater. It is composed of elastic and collagenous fibers, arranged in seemingly disorganized crisscrossed clusters. In fact, the fibers are arranged in concentric layers. Orientation of fibers varies from one layer to the next, but is consistent (usually longitudinal) within a given layer.

The thickness of the dura mater depends upon its location *(Fig. 2-6)*:

- foramen magnum to C3: 0.68mm
- cervicothoracic region: 0.50mm
- lumbosacral region: 0.73–0.33mm
- medullary cone: 0.33mm.

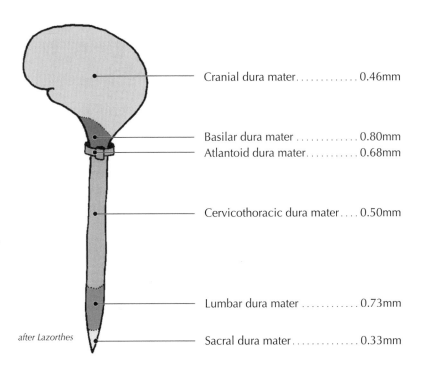

Cranial dura mater 0.46mm

Basilar dura mater 0.80mm
Atlantoid dura mater 0.68mm

Cervicothoracic dura mater 0.50mm

Lumbar dura mater 0.73mm

Sacral dura mater 0.33mm

after Lazorthes

Fig. 2-6: Variations in the width of the dura mater (average values)

DURA MATER ATTACHMENTS

Upper attachments
- The spinal dura mater is continuous with the cranial dura mater at the level of the foramen magnum periphery, to which it adheres by a strong fibrous band.
- It is attached to the posterior surface of the body of the axis.

Lower attachments
- Throughout the length of the dural cul-de-sac (the summit of which corresponds to S2) the fibrous extensions between the anterior face of the dura mater and the common posterior vertebral ligament grow and thicken to form Trolard's sacrodural ligament.
- The lower edge of the dural cul-de-sac tapers to adhere to the coccyx and form the durococcygeal ligament.

Lateral attachments
- The dura mater is contiguous with the epineureum and the dentate ligaments.

Anterior attachments
- The dura mater is attached to the common posterior vertebral ligament by several fibrous extensions.

IMPORTANT LIGAMENTOUS RELATIONSHIPS

- Common posterior vertebral ligament. This separates from the basilar groove anterior to the foramen magnum and merges anteriorly with the apical ligament of dens. It is attached to the posterior part of the vertebral bodies, in the middle of the spinal canal. It is narrower at the level of the vertebral bodies, and wider at the level of the disks, to which it adheres closely. Its posterior surface is attached to the dura mater by connective tissue tracts.
- Sacrodural ligament. This is a part of the common posterior vertebral ligament, and joins the dura mater to the anterior wall of the sacral canal. The common posterior vertebral ligament tapers below the lumbosacral joint, ending on the first coccygeal segment. The deep portion of the posterior sacrococcygeal ligament corresponds to the common posterior vertebral ligament.
- Ligamentum flavum. The anterior surface of this interlamellar ligament corresponds to the spinal dura mater, from which it is separated by fat and veins of the spinal cord.
- Posterior occipitoaxial ligament. Perforations on the right and left permit the passage of the vertebral arteries and the first cervical nerve. Represents a combination of the tectorial membrane and the alar ligaments.
- Apical ligament of dens. Its posterior part corresponds to the common posterior vertebral ligament.

VERTEBRAL FORAMEN

Three elements are closely connected in the vertebral foramen: the roots and spinal ganglion, fat, and veins. In principle, the dural radicular adipose tissue and its swelling at the level of the ganglion are not attached at the level of the vertebral foramen.

Cervical level

The orifice is extended by the transverse fissure to which the perineurium of the cervical nerves are adherent. The vertebral foramen is comprised of two parts:

- the posteromedial part, or vertebral foramen proper
- the anterolateral part, or transverse fissure, perforated at the bottom by the orifice of the vertebral artery.

Cervical disk hernias are often found laterally just behind the junction of the main vertebral body and the raised lip on its upper surface (also known as the uncinate process). These can cause venous stasis, edema, and direct compression of the roots and ganglia.

Some osteopaths obtain rapid results with cervicobrachial neuralgias and sciaticas using techniques which promote drainage of periradicular edema resulting from venous stasis.

Lumbar level

The nerves are situated on the upper part of the foramen, which serves as a protective barrier against variations in height due to disk compression and mobility of the posterior articular processes. The two or three sensory roots are posterior, and the anterior root is superior and forward. Fat supports and protects the nerve alignments. The nerve roots are also protected by fibrous adherence of the perineurium to the walls of the transverse foraminal channel.

Conclusion

At the spinal level, attention to several attachments of the dura mater is required for successful osteopathic manipulation:

- foramen magnum
- C2
- sacrum
- coccyx
- vertebral foramen.

Dura mater of the craniospinal junction

The two germ layers of the cranial dura mater, until now joined together, separate in the spinal canal and define the epidural space:

- the external germ layer (periosteal layer) joins the canal walls
- the internal germ layer continues as the spinal dura mater.

According to Lazorthes (1953), the posterior occipitoatloid and atloaxoid ligaments are not really ligamentous elements, but rather a periosteal continuation of the occipital and the intraspinal periosteum attached to the dura mater *(Fig. 2-7)*.

The high mobility of C1 results in formation of a space between the two dura mater germ layers. In flexion-extension movements, the posterior dura mater of C1 stretches and relaxes, causing opening and closing of the interdural space.

Laterally, the craniospinal dura mater participates in formation of the sheath for the vertebral artery. At the exit of the transverse canal of C1, horizontally, the vertebral artery is located between the periosteum of the occipital bone and the sheath formed by C1.

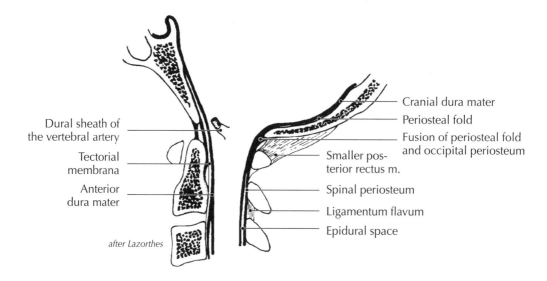

Fig. 2-7: Dura mater of the craniospinal juncture (sagittal section)

The artery reaches the dura mater, crosses it, compresses it, and carries it in the spinal canal in a sort of sheath which continues for several millimeters before slowly merging with its adventitia *(Fig. 2-8)*.

Anteriorly, the dura mater is very thick, and closely adheres to:

- the tectorial membrane and alar ligaments
- the basilar groove anterior to the foramen magnum
- the rim of the foramen magnum
- the contours of the top of the odontoid process.

Below this last structure, the adhesion stops and the epidural space begins.

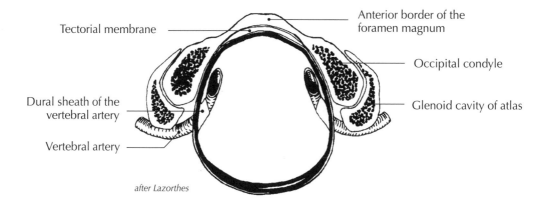

Fig. 2-8: Dura mater of the craniospinal juncture
(oblique section at level of foramen magnum)

CRANIAL DURA MATER

The cranial dura mater constitutes a hollow sphere which envelops the mass of the brain. It also lines the cranial cavity, for which it serves as an internal periosteum

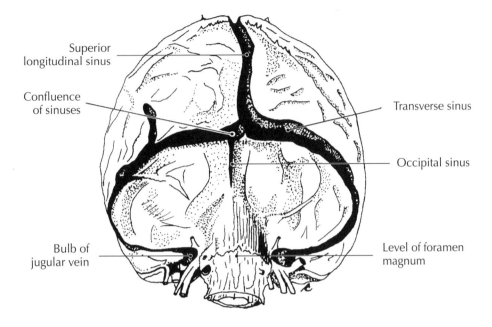

Fig. 2-9: Separate posterior view of the dura mater surrounding the encephalon

(Fig. 2-9).

External surface

The external surface of the cranial dura mater faces the internal wall of the skull, to which it is attached by fibrous and vascular extensions. It is weakly adherent to the vault, except at the level of the sutures. As a child grows, adherence to the cranial cavity increases with age due to density of the fibrous tracts which run from the membrane to the bones, and encrustations of the arachnoidal granulations.

Adherence of the dura mater is more marked in a child than in an adult. The dura mater of an infant detaches with difficulty during trauma, and tears at the level of the fracture. The dura mater sheaths surrounding the cranial nerves strengthen adherence of the dura mater to the base of the skull. The two germ layers of the dura mater are joined in the adult, and divide at the foramen magnum to descend separately into the spinal canal, as described above.

Strong attachments of the cranial dura mater

- base of skull (primarily the crista galli)
- posterior edge of the lesser sphenoid wings
- anterior and posterior clinoid processes
- upper edge of petrous bone

- basilar groove anterior to foramen magnum
- rim of foramen magnum.

Internal surface

The three intracranial septa of the dura mater *(Fig. 2-10)* are well known in osteopathy. Their primary role is to isolate and stabilize the various parts of the brain in all positions, during direct or indirect trauma. They are:

- falx cerebri
- tentorium cerebelli
- falx cerebelli

Despite being firmly stabilized, the brain can still be mobilized in the cranial cavity during trauma, as discussed previously. Anteroposterior movements are the most common.

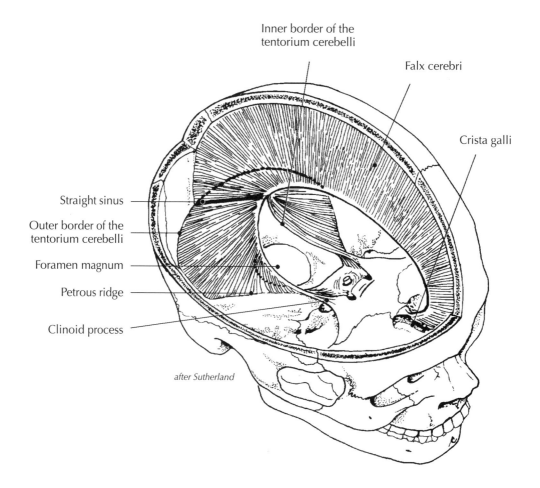

Fig. 2-10: Intracranial reciprocal tension membranes

Neuromeningeal dynamics

Movements of the nervous system, although initially difficult to detect, do exist. Not all can be demonstrated by current imaging methods, but some have been quantified.

Many studies have focused on how trauma affects the dynamics of the brain and spinal cord. It is clear that, at least in certain regions of the CNS, there are movements of neurological "content" which differ from those of the osteomeningeal "container." On the basis of studies by Breig (1978), Louis (1981), and Rabischong (1989), with comparison to histological analysis, we shall now consider:

- the concept of visceral articulation and how it applies to the CNS
- the surfaces involved in this articulation
- means of connection and limitation of movement
- physiology of movement
- pathophysiological mechanics.

Visceral articulation

CONCEPT OF NEURAL OSTEOMENINGEAL ARTICULATION

We described previously the concept of visceral articulation in the thoracic and abdominopelvic compartments (Barral & Mercier, 1988). Sliding surfaces are formed by serous membranes, lubricated by serous fluid. The spaces formed, which are closed on all sides, have a resemblance to joint capsules and permit movement through sliding of the visceral structures.

In this case, the analogy with osteoarticular joints is fairly easy to establish. We should note that the functional classification of joints includes the *syssarcosis*, which is an articulation made up of muscles. This category can logically be extended to include visceral articulations, that is, sliding surfaces such as the serous synovial bursae, tendinous synovial sheaths, and other fibrous structures that facilitate movement.

The "articular" analogy is more difficult to defend in terms of the differential movements of the CNS relative to its bony container. Histologically speaking, contrary to general belief, the nervous system's envelopes do not contain serous membranes. Also, the sliding requirements differ from those of body viscera. They are related primarily to the vulnerability of nervous tissues to compression stress and the need to be protected. Movement of CNS structures does occur, and the features permitting it, even if biomechanically different from those of body visceral articulations, are real and well-adapted to their function.

COMMON MENINGEAL STRUCTURES

The neural tissue of the CNS is covered by a meningeal system which follows its contours closely *(Fig. 2-11)*. The pia mater constitutes the internal or "visceral" portion of the sliding system. The "parietal" portion consists of:

- an external layer, the dura mater, which is membranous, resistant, not very extendible, and which lines the internal surface of the osseous "container"
- an intermediate layer, the arachnoid, a connective tissue membrane without vessels or nerves. It lines the deep surface of the dura mater and has connective fiber attachments to the pia mater.

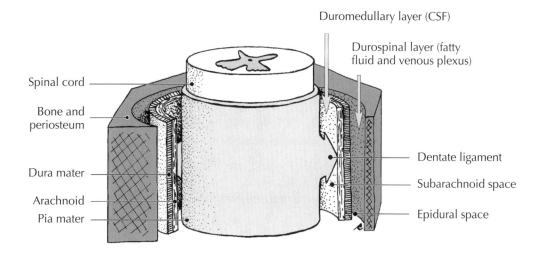

Fig. 2-11: Medullospinal articular surfaces

The subarachnoid space, between the arachnoid and pia mater, is the external fluid compartment of the CNS. This space is filled with CSF, and has multiple functions—one of which is mobilization of one surface in relation to the other.

EPIDURAL SPACE

This space, situated between the dura mater and the osteofibrous walls of the spinal canal, is virtual. It is occupied primarily by adipose tissue and the network of epidural veins comprising the intraspinal plexus. The space is actually formed by a doubling of the dura mater tissue, which is histologically composed of two layers.

- At the cranial level, these two layers are joined together. The external layer functions as an endocranial periosteum, and the internal layer as a vessel carrier.
- At the upper spinal level, these two layers separate. The external layer functions as periosteum inside the spinal canal, and the internal layer constitutes the spinal dura mater proper. Together, they delimit the epidural space.

Rabischong (1989) attributes a double function to the epidural space:

- to promote the mechanical adaptation between the vertebral canal and dural sheath
- to serve as a medium of venous circulation with hemopoietic function, starting from the spongy tissue of the vertebral body.

This additional sliding surface is a flexible interface which is not very confining. Nonetheless, it permits stabilization of the duromedullary element, while reducing the influence of the osteofibrous element in the vertebral canal.

MEANS OF CONNECTION

In our articular model of the CNS, there are two types of connection between adjacent structures:

- physiological effects, which increase cohesion between container and content, or reduce the effective weight of a visceral structure
- anatomic structures. Some of these, such as the dura mater, are strongly constructed. Others may appear weaker, but are still well-adapted to their particular mechanical environment.

TURGOR EFFECT

This physical effect, related to splanchnic visceral turgidity, has an equivalent at the level of the CNS, primarily the brain. Increased requirements for nutrients (sugar and oxygen) require optimal blood perfusion of the encephalic structures. As in the vessels of the kidney, pressure in the arterial trunks which supply the brain is of primary importance for maintaining constant pressure and rate of cerebral blood flow.

Under the effect of the arterial blood pressure, the brain tends to occupy all the space made available to it, with limits imposed by the volume of the cranial cavity and the CSF in which it is bathed. Since the CNS is not tolerant of compression, the sum of the volumes of the nervous tissue, CSF, and local blood mass must be maintained at a nearly constant level.

Perfusion pressure and the geometry of the arteries contribute to expansion of the cerebral tissue. All the blood vessels enter the cranium at the base, and the forces of turgidity spread out in a multidirectional manner toward the cranial vault. The fact that the cerebral mass is bathed on all sides by CSF further enhances this effect. This turgor effect seems to create a flower-like "blossoming" of the cerebral mass. It is a significant factor limiting the effective weight of the brain.

CSF PRESSURE

One function of the CSF, discussed previously, is to protect the CNS from trauma via its hydraulic dampening capacity. CSF hydrodynamics can be studied by measuring CSF pressure during a lumbar puncture. This pressure is ~120mm H_2O in a supine subject. We assume that normal CSF pressure is below 200mm H_2O at lumbar level in supine position (or at foramen magnum level in seated position).

The CSF has a pressure gradient which depends on the position of the subject. Hydrostatic pressure is highest in the "lowest" parts of the system. For example:

- pressure in supine position at the lumbar level: 100 to 150mm H_2O
- pressure in seated position at the lumbar level: 200 to 300mm H_2O

CSF pressure is subject to numerous sources of variation:

- it increases in response to abdominal pressure
- it is not influenced by changes in arterial pressure, but is extremely sensitive to changes in level of carbon dioxide (hyperventilation decreases intracranial pressure) and venous pressure
- it increases in response to jugular vein compression.

The Queckenstedt-Stookey test, designed to reveal such variations, examines changes in CSF pressure over 5-second intervals, in response to a 20-second compression of the jugular vein. Return to normal usually occurs within 20 seconds after compression ceases.

ARCHIMEDEAN THRUST

The entire CNS, bathing in the fluid volume of the CSF, is subject to Archimedes' principle. This stipulates that all diving bodies, whether floating or submerged in a fluid, are subject to an upwardly directed force or *Archimedean thrust*. The thrust exerted on the body is equal to the weight of the displaced fluid.

Livingston's (1965) work demonstrated that the entire CNS receives such a thrust, which considerably reduces effective weight because of the low overall density of the CNS. The thrust induced by the CSF is such that a brain weighing 1500g in air weighs only 50g relative to its attachments when submerged in CSF *in situ*.

The effect of this Archimedean thrust on the statics of the CNS explains, in our opinion, why any decrease in CSF volume has such clinical significance. If fluid volume decreases, the Archimedean thrust also decreases, thereby increasing the effective over-all weight of the CNS. This increase in weight overloads other methods of connection and support, creating tensions and irritations throughout the meningeal system. In particularly severe cases, the increase in effective weight of the brain results in contact of neural tissues with bony tissue of the foramen magnum.

DURA MATER ATTACHMENTS

There are numerous anatomic and mechanical distinctions between the cranial and spinal segments of the dura mater.

The anchoring of the dura mater to the internal surface of its bony container does not constitute a method of connection for visceral articulation, but is nonetheless important for the statics and dynamics of this system.

In the skull, the most important anchors of the dura mater are at the contoured areas of the base and the level of the craniocervical hinge. At the spinal level the only true fixed point of the dura mater is at the sacrum, and to a lesser extent the base of the coccyx. There are sometimes attachments to the body of C2 and/or C3.

EPIDURAL "SUCTION"

The epidural space is an area of negative pressure, a fact useful for anesthesiologists giving epidural anesthesia. The suction effect permits them to locate the proper injection depth for the anesthetic using a technique referred to as the "hanging drop": a drop of liquid anesthetic applied to the base of the needle is aspirated when it penetrates into the dural space. The negative pressure in the epidural space grants it a certain stability, despite its lack of vertebral attachments.

We believe that this relative stability in the absence of a ligamentous type of anatomical substrate permits permanent adaptation of the contents to the container, in accordance with the dynamic or static factors of the spine. We also believe that it plays an important role, through its effect as a vacuum cup, on the turgidity of the duromedullary sheath.

This "vacuum" effect contributes to a degree of "prestressing through inflation," that is, the hydrostatic pressure of the CSF is reinforced by epidural suction. This permanent prestressing provides good mechanical resistance to lateral compression stress, which is especially dangerous for the spinal cord. Epidural suction also plays an important role in intraspinal venous circulation by promoting opening of the epidural veins.

INTRACRANIAL DURA MATER STRUCTURES

The falx cerebri, falx cerebelli, and tentorium cerebelli divide the cranial cavity into four subcavities. These meningeal structures are referred to by osteopaths as reciprocal tension membranes.

We envision these dura mater structures in the context of statics and dynamics at the level of macroscopic movement, and define them as agents of equilibration and protection in the CNS.

These membranes play a major role in visceral articulation through the support they provide to various encephalic regions. They keep the brain optimally centered in the three dimensions of the cranial cavity. Through the divisions they impose upon the brain and external fluid compartment, they reduce stresses on the brain by dividing Archimedean thrust as evenly as possible. The presence of deep clefts permits this division of fluid to the deepest recesses of the encephalic masses.

ROOTS, NERVES, AND VERTEBRAL FORAMEN

Nerve roots throughout the summit of the medulla oblongata and spinal cord are grouped in a series of small roots from which the cranial and spinal nerves originate. All these nerve outgrowths constitute potential fixed or semifixed points *(Fig. 2-12)*.

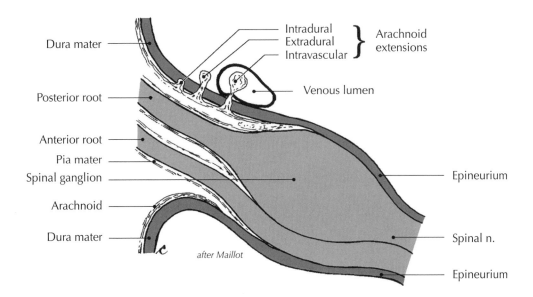

Fig. 2-12: Relationship between the meninges and nerve roots

The nerves play an important mechanical role due to the meningeal continuity on their coverings, and the different structures which attach them to the vertebral foramen. Stresses exerted via the nerves can create or limit CNS movement.

DENTATE LIGAMENTS

On each lateral fasciculus, equidistant from the anterior and posterior roots, is a thin, fibrous septum called the dentate ligament. These digitations, averaging 21 teeth on each side, are spread over the height of the spinal cord. They are flexible links stretching between the pia mater and the deep surface of the spinal dura mater. They resemble the pia mater in its medial and dural parts, relative to its free edge. At the edge of each tooth, the dentate ligament is progressively indistinguishable from the inner layers of the dura mater *(Fig. 2-13)*.

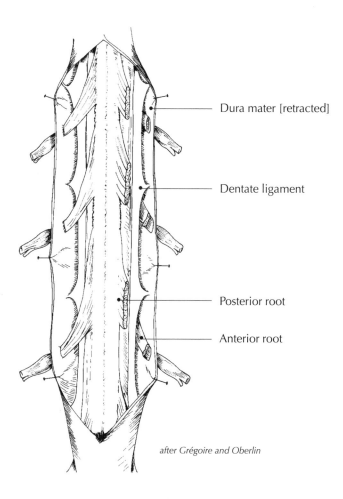

Dura mater [retracted]

Dentate ligament

Posterior root

Anterior root

after Grégoire and Oberlin

Fig. 2-13: The dura mater and spinal roots

The dentate ligament essentially suspends the spinal cord inside its dural case. It ensures dynamic centering of the spinal cord in the spinal canal, in all positions and for all spinal movements. Its role for the spinal cord is like that of the falx cerebri and tentorium cerebelli for the brain.

ARACHNOID TRABECULAE

The arachnoid trabeculae constitute small bridges between the dura mater and pia mater, and help anchor the CNS to the interior of the dura mater. They also divide the subarachnoid space into distinct fluid cells, causing it to function like a sheet of bubble wrap, with CSF substituting for air. This method of connection is probably essentially static and appropriate for brief, mild applied force. It does not provide protection against major mechanical CNS stress, as during trauma.

Physiology of Movement

The spinal cord and spinal canal

The spinal cord does not extend farther than L2. The disparity in length between dura mater and spinal cord is easily explained embryologically. In the fetus, the spinal cord descends until the lower part of the sacral canal. However, osseous growth occurs in a more consistent way and more rapidly than neural growth. As the embryo continues growing, the medullary cone of the spinal cord ascends relative to the osteodural case.

Comparison of the spinal cord and canal

One of the primary roles of the vertebral column is to protect the spinal cord while allowing movement at the level of the brainstem. The spinal canal is a long, irregularly shaped osteofibrous tunnel which follows the spinal curvature. Its diameter varies depending on spinal level. It closely follows variations in diameter of the spinal cord. It is widest at the cervical and lumbar level, and narrowest at the level of T4 and T6 *(Fig. 2-*

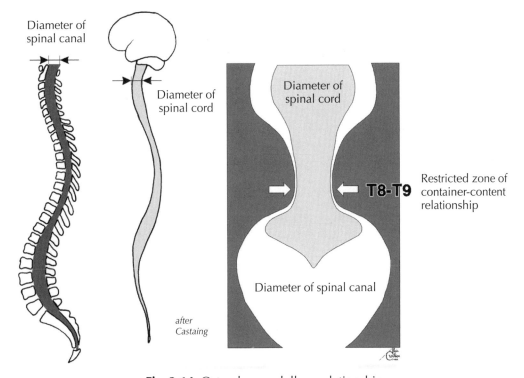

Fig. 2-14: Osteoduromedullary relationship

14). However, diameters of the spinal cord and spinal canal do not vary in strict parallel, that is, adaptation of container to contents is not complete:

- at the lumbar and cervical levels, the spinal cord is relatively large in the spinal canal

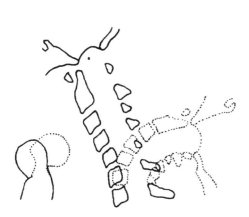

Fig. 2-15: Variations in length of the cervical canal during flexion and extension of the neck

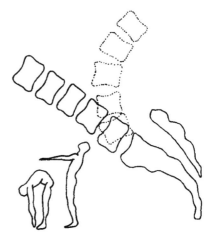

Fig. 2-16: Variations in length of the lumbar canal during flexion and extension of the trunk

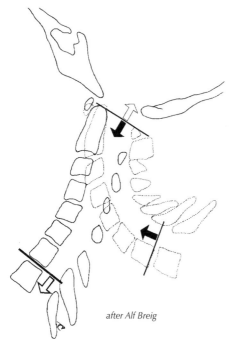

after Alf Breig

Diagram composed by superposition of two x-rays, with the base of the skull as a point of reference. In flexion the cervical canal is stretched; it is shortened in extension. The posterior wall of the canal is more affected by the change in length. In the case shown, there is a variation of approximately 3cm in the middle of the canal.

Fig. 2-17: The cervical canal in full flexion and extension

• at the lower thoracic level, the spinal cord is very narrow in the spinal canal, particularly at T8 and T9.

Spinal canal and spinal mechanics

The dimensions of the spinal canal vary greatly along its length and between flexion and extension, particularly in the cervical and lumbar regions *(Figs. 2-15 to 2-17).*

	Flexion (in mm)	Extension (in mm)
Cervical spine	+ 28	- 15
Dorsal spine	+ 3	- 3
Lumbar spine	+ 28	- 20

Table 2-1: Segmental variations in length of the vertebral canal (source: P. Rabischong)

According to some authors, these changes are on the order of 5 to 9cm.

The intervertebral spaces are greatly stretched in their posterior section during spinal hyperflexion, and contracted during hyperextension. It is not hard to understand how the vertebral canal can lengthen by as much as 9cm during spinal hyperflexion, relative to the position of extension, in young and flexible subjects. Similarly, in side-

	Weight (in g)	Relationship between spinal cord / element considered
Spinal cord	27	-
Isthmus and bulb	26	1/1
Cerebellum	140	1/5
Brain	1170	1/43
Encephalon	1358	1/48

Table 2-2: Respective weights and proportions of the different segments of the central nervous system

bending, the canal lengthens convexly and shortens concavely. These variations in length are significant at the cervical and lumbar levels, but slight at the thoracic level *(Table 2-1).*

Statics of the spinal cord

The spinal cord is firmer than the brain or cerebellum, due to a thick layer of peripheral white matter. The absolute weight of the spinal cord, without spinal roots and nerves, is 26-30g in men, 24-28g in women. The following table, modified from Testut, shows weights of the different segments of the CNS *(Table 2-2)*.

The spinal cord weighs 48 times less than the brain. The medulla oblongata and spinal cord have a combined weight of only ~55g. The spinal cord must therefore draw on stabilizing elements in order for the cerebrospinal group to remain in equilibrium. Otherwise, it would have to endure all the distortions imposed by the brain during acceleration, changes in position, and bodily movements.

The spinal cord is not simply a "large nerve," as stated by some early anatomists. Although it certainly plays the role of conductor, it also represents a nerve control and distribution center with its white matter (myelinated axons). The latter function must receive appropriate mechanical protection. In our opinion, the filum terminale plays a mechanical role much more important than generally believed. Through this caudad attachment, the spinal cord is prestressed with tension, and not mechanically locked to the encephalic mass.

The position of the neural axis changes according to the subject's position.

- Spinal extension: the spinal cord is shortened and presses against the posterior wall of the spinal canal.
- Spinal flexion: the spinal cord is in tension and presses against the anterior wall of the spinal canal.
- Supine position: subject to the effect of gravity, the spinal cord is closer to the posterior wall of the spinal canal. The brain presses toward the occipital part of the skull, and the anterior arachnoid structures are tractioned.
- Prone position: the spinal cord is close to the anterior wall of the spinal canal. The brain presses toward the frontal part of the skull, and the posterior arachnoid structures are tractioned.

Dynamics of the cord and vertebrae

The spinal cord, roots, and meningeal envelopes must stretch or shorten in response to changes in length of the vertebral canal *(Figs. 2-18 & 2-19)*. At its cranial end, the spinal dura mater is attached to the circumference of the foramen magnum; at its caudad edge, it is moored to the sacrococcyx by the sacrodural ligament and filum terminale.

- During full extension, the spinal cord is slightly folded and increases in thickness at the expense of its length, which decreases without axial sliding *(Fig. 2-19)*.
- During full flexion of the brainstem, the dura mater is under tension, like the spinal cord. Part of this medullary tension is due to transmission of dura mater stress to the pia mater, via the dentate ligaments (which keep the spinal cord as frontally centered as possible). However, the greatest tension is applied directly to the spinal cord, because it is anchored to the two edges by the cerebral peduncles and cauda equina.

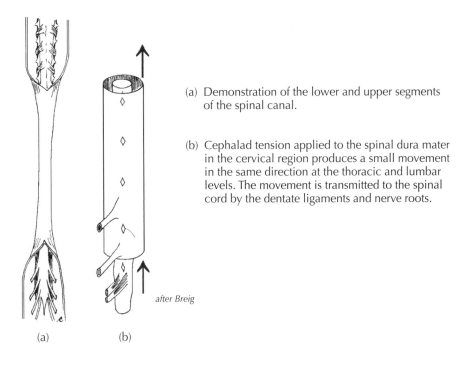

(a) Demonstration of the lower and upper segments of the spinal canal.

(b) Cephalad tension applied to the spinal dura mater in the cervical region produces a small movement in the same direction at the thoracic and lumbar levels. The movement is transmitted to the spinal cord by the dentate ligaments and nerve roots.

after Breig

(a)   (b)

Fig. 2-18: Transmission of tension in the spinal dura mater

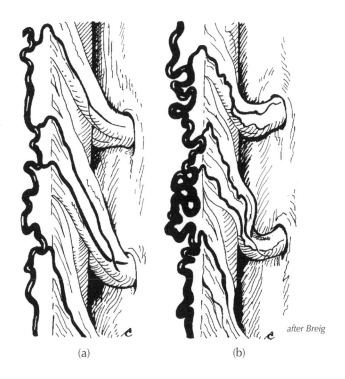

after Breig

(a)   (b)

Fig. 2-19: Cervical cord during flexion (a) and extension (b) of the neck

Concept of the "pons-cord tract"

We agree with Breig that the spinal cord cannot be studied biomechanically in isolation; rather, it should be considered as a continuous tract of nervous and support tissue, stretching from the mesencephalon to the medullary cone and cauda equina. Breig refers to this entity as the pons-cord tract (PCT).

The static and dynamic properties of this tract facilitate understanding of the effects of trauma, and a global view of cranial/spinal mechanics.

- During spinal extension, from a neutral position, the axes of the spinal canal and PCT are shortened, and the tissues are relaxed and folded *(Fig. 2-20)*.
- In neutral position, the PCT regains its original length, relaxation ceases, and the folds are eliminated.
- In flexion, during which the spinal canal increases in length, the PCT is stretched.

During these spinal movements, the axons and blood vessels undergo distortion similar to that of the PCT.

Even though the dura mater is fixed at the base of the skull and sacrum, these attachments should not be confused with those of the PCT. Distally, the PCT is moored

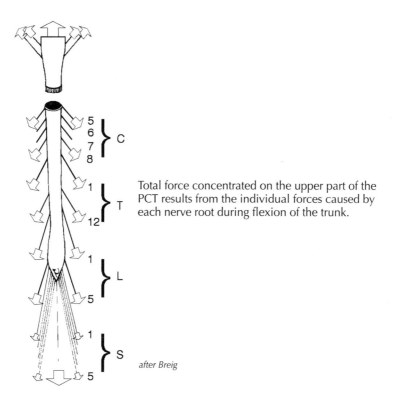

Total force concentrated on the upper part of the PCT results from the individual forces caused by each nerve root during flexion of the trunk.

after Breig

Fig. 2-20: Increase in cephalad traction with spinal flexion

by the roots and cauda equina at the lumbar vertebral foramina and sacral foramina, and by the filum terminale at the base of the coccyx.

During spinal flexion movements, tension of the roots and filum is communicated to the spinal cord. This is particularly marked near the cauda equina, where forces converge toward the medullary cone to stretch it. To a lesser extent, the other spinal roots also contribute to the stretching of the PCT, but stretching by the distal roots is due primarily to their number and vertical orientation. Distal tension increases progressively up to the top of the spinal cord and pontine region *(Fig. 2-20)*.

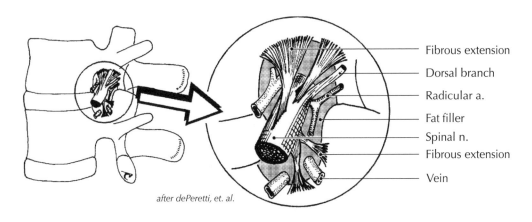

after dePeretti, et. al.

Fig. 2-21: Lateral view of the intervertebral foramen with the ateriovenous, adipose, and fibrous elements

Intervertebral foramen

Studies by de Peretti in Nice demonstrated the error of the conventional description of the intervertebral foramen as closed off by a membrane stretched like a drumskin. The nerve root is, in fact, attached to the foramen by many piercing extensions *(Fig. 2-21)*.

Specifically, there are two sites of nerve and root fixation:

- the radicular neck of the dura mater
- numerous fibrous extensions at the periphery of the foramen.

Nerve sheaths

In a section of a spinal nerve the continuity between the medullary envelopes and the nerve sheaths is obvious. The dura mater joins the epineurium without any break. Laterally, the arachnoid accompanies the nerve roots in the dural sheaths. In the area of the radicular angle, the subarachnoid space disappears as the pia mater and arachnoid are joined together, then merge with the nerve sheath itself *(Figs. 2-22 & 2-23)*.

According to Rabischong, there is a "stacked binding" along the length of the epineurium from a given connective space. This explains how a fluid introduced in the subarachnoid space spreads throughout the nerve sheath. Resorption of CSF occurs at

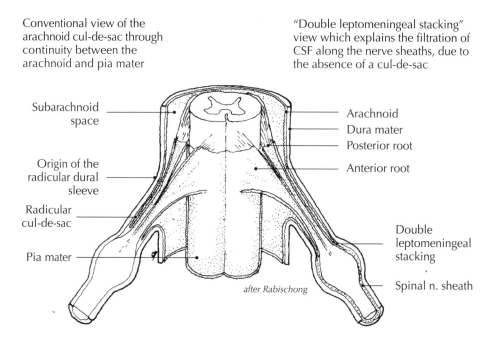

Conventional view of the arachnoid cul-de-sac through continuity between the arachnoid and pia mater

"Double leptomeningeal stacking" view which explains the filtration of CSF along the nerve sheaths, due to the absence of a cul-de-sac

Subarachnoid space

Arachnoid
Dura mater
Posterior root

Origin of the radicular dural sleeve

Anterior root

Radicular cul-de-sac

Double leptomeningeal stacking

Pia mater

Spinal n. sheath

after Rabischong

Fig. 2-22: Organization of the spinal meninges

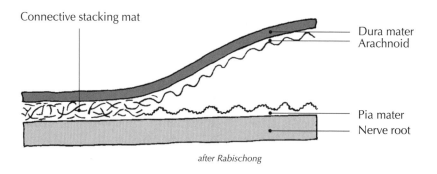

Connective stacking mat

Dura mater
Arachnoid

Pia mater
Nerve root

after Rabischong

Fig. 2-23: Detail of double leptomeningeal stacking

the level of this connective stacking, which complements the resorption in the arachnoidal granulations, ensuring complete CSF recirculation four times per day. However, the process is one of diffusion and current-induced circulation, similar to the encephalic ventricular system.

Nerve roots

The roots originate at the lateral sulci of the spinal cord. The anterior roots have a common origin, while the posterior roots originate from a series of four to eight rootlets which then reunite to form one or several radicular fascicles. The orientation of roots follows the progressive staggering of myelomere levels.

Below the medullary cone, the vertebral canal is occupied exclusively by the vertical lumbosacral roots, which join together as the cauda equina around the filum terminale. Roots in the cervical area are slightly oblique. Horizontally, orientation also

Traction (in g)	Displacement (in mm)
50	0
500	0.5
1,000	1
1,500	1
2,000	2
2,500	2.5
3,000	3

Table 2-3: Relationship of lumbar root traction / displacement (after De Perett et al.)

varies depending on vertebral level. These orientations affect the statics and dynamics of roots and nerves at different levels. The vertical lumbosacral roots experience most of the stress imposed by the PCT.

Study of root mobility reveals the existence of two distinct compartments: intraspinal and extraspinal. The foraminal attachments constitute a barrier between the two compartments, such that movements imposed on one are not felt in the other. The fibrous barriers stop the movement imposed upon the spinal nerve, outside the intervertebral foramen. The intervertebral foramen seems to act as a major barrier for tension imposed from outside the spinal canal. De Peretti demonstrated that under significant traction the nerves and roots do exhibit slight mobility. Results of tests of dynamometric traction are shown in Table 2-3.

During spinal movement, flexion and sidebending stress the PCT and create tension on the nerve roots. Maximal physiological tension experienced by the lumbar roots is ~100g. Think of what this could mean for a nerve composed of rootlets.

These results imply that during normal spinal and pelvic movements, tension applied to the lumbar roots does not cause significant nerve mobility outside the intervertebral foramen. This confirms the resistance of the foraminal attachments to weak tension, and demonstrates the necessity of some normal slack available to the rootlets.

Significant forces of traction can act upon the intervertebral foramen, in addition to the stretching of the elements focused on the nerve and dural sheath. Nerve protection is afforded primarily by three factors:

- the normal slack of the roots through the dura mater, which prevents development of tension independent of movement
- the hydraulic compartment created by the CSF

• clustering of local adipose tissue and epidural venous plexuses.

Spinal cord dynamics

It is surprising that nervous tissue can be a vector for mechanical strains.

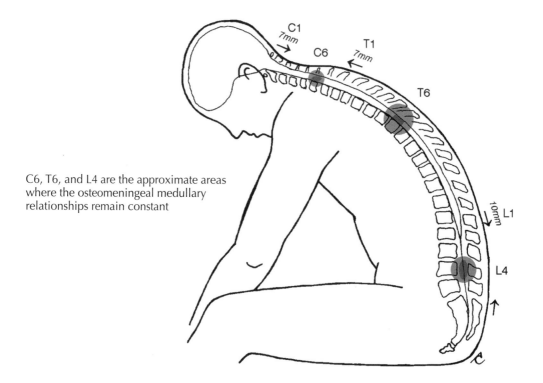

C6, T6, and L4 are the approximate areas where the osteomeningeal medullary relationships remain constant

Fig. 2-24: Medullary dynamics during spinal flexion

Although often viewed as fragile or delicate, it has great mechanical resistance. Its capacity to endure stress in traction during spinal movements suggested to us the potential role of such stimulation for metabolic and physiological purposes.

During forced spinal flexion, the various segments of the spinal column, like those of the spinal dura mater, are displaced axially toward the most mobile cervical (C6) and lumbar (L4) vertebra *(Fig. 2-24)*. Osteomeningomedullary relationships remain unchanged.

• Regions of greatest axial spinal cord displacement relative to the walls of the vertebral canal are around C1 (7mm, caudad), T1 (7mm, cranially), and L1 (10mm, caudad).
• The regions of minimal (almost no) sliding are at the top of the cervical lordosis (C6) and the thoracic kyphosis (T6).

In addition to axial sliding due to stretching of the spinal cord, there are regions whose tension varies with the myelomeres. Two spinal cord regions, the lower parts of the cervical (C6 to T2) and lumbar (L4 to coccyx) enlargements, are particularly involved in stretching. The former region corresponds to the region of greatest cervical mobility (C5-T1). The latter region is explained by transmission to the medullary cone of the forces of stretching controlling the lumbosacral roots underlying L4.

The total degree of possible stretching of the spinal cord is roughly a tenth of its length, that is, 43mm in a spinal cord 43cm long. The vertebral canal is lengthened by 59mm going from straight (neutral) position to hyperflexion. This lengthening is not equally distributed, that is, some regions undergo stretching equal to a fifth of their initial length, whereas the thoracic region hardly stretches at all.

According to Louis (1981), in hyperflexion, neurological lesions may occur at the level of the cervical and lumbar enlargements by a simple exaggeration of this maximal tension. These lesions may result in quadriplegia or paraplegia, depending upon the level affected, even in the absence of osseous injury. This probably explains some of the neurological lesions following spinal trauma in which no osseous lesions appear on imaging studies. These are similar to brachial plexus lesions.

The bulbar, cervical, and lumbar enlargements effectively constitute a "reserve" of nervous tissue when the spine is straight or extended. These segments are easily stretched during spinal flexion.

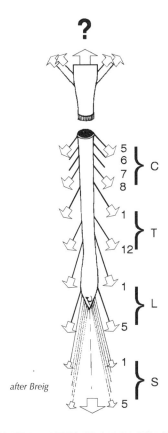

Fig. 2-25: Traction forces on the spinal cord

Statics and dynamics of the CNS

Role of the tentorium cerebelli

Breig made a diagram of the forces of traction on the spinal cord *(Fig. 2-25)*. Looking at this, we wondered how the distal tension is counterbalanced. The laws of equilibrium require that every force have an equilibrating force. In our case, equilibration cannot be due to pressing of the medulla oblongata or cerebellum on the rim of the foramen magnum. These structures are much too vulnerable to the danger of compression stress.

Even though the osteoarticular junction between the skull and spine occurs at the level of the occipitoatloid interarticular space, the mechanical junction between spinal cord and encephalon is not at the same spot. The cranial portion of the PCT is not moored to the occiput by the cerebellum, as we might assume. It has very little relationship with this bone. Anatomic dampening and protective structures (CSF cisternae at the level of the skull and medulla oblongata; position of spinal cord and medulla in the foramen magnum) argue in favor of another type of PCT suspension. In fact, the upper suspension of the PCT is provided by the cranial nerves and the anchoring of the isthmus of the encephalon in the diencephalic mass. This poses a question: Why does cerebral engagement not occur every time the spine is significantly flexed?

There are several elements that oppose this tendency: arachnoid trabeculations attaching the brain to the dura mater of the vault, environmental fluid pressure, turgor effect from perfusion pressure of the encephalon. However, only one structure is mechanically capable of opposing such a connection: the *tentorium cerebelli*. This scrupulously circumscribes the region of the cerebral peduncles, at its lesser circumference, and supports the entire posterior section of the brain in the posterior cranial fossa.

The tentorium indirectly suspends the entire spinal cord and medulla oblongata. It dampens the tensions caused by vertebral mechanics, by opposing distal traction operating on the PCT. This horizontal structure of the tentorium is suspended from a vertical structure, the *falx cerebri*, and is thus not only moored to the contours of the base of the skull, but also suspended from the calvaria.

The PCT is suspended flexibly from the tentorium cerebelli, creating an actual pocket which supports the telencephalic mass. The PCT is subjected to tension depending upon spinal movements and postures.

Since the tentorium cerebelli is attached to the falx cerebri, any stress affecting the tentorium has repercussions on the falx via traction. The "dense" attachments of the intracranial dura mater are also involved. Moreover, since the tentorium supports the brain, any strong mechanical stress disturbs this fragile cerebropontomedullary equilibrium.

Collectively, the intracranial membranes can be compared to a three-dimensional trampoline, or a mushroom with two heads and one foot. The foot of the mushroom passes through the opening of the trampoline. We can see how the entire neural axis is suspended by reciprocal tension membranes *(Fig. 2-26)*. Under such conditions, any stress on the foot also involves the head, pocket, and its entire system of attachments.

This model helps us visualize how neuromeningeal dynamics constitute an inseparable whole, and why certain types of "whiplash" involve the entire craniosacral system in addition to vertebral mechanics. Conversely, in pathological conditions such as certain types of scoliosis, disturbances of tension in the intracranial membranes can negatively impact vertebral mechanics.

Intracranial membranes

In view of the above relationships, we can see that:

- spinal flexion pulls on the PCT, and the encephalon lowers the tentorium cere-

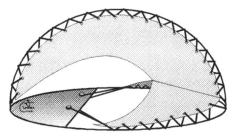

The intracranial membranes may be compared to a perforated three-dimensional trampoline which overhangs the posterior cerebral fossa.

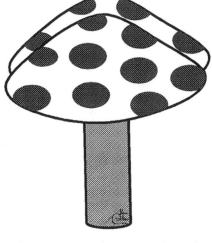

The neuraxis can be compared to a "bi-cephalic" mushroom: the foot represents the PCT and the two hats represent the cerebral hemispheres.

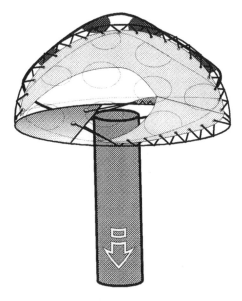

The entire device in place. The hats are on the trampoline, the foot passes through the perforation (homologous with the free edge of the tentorium cerebelli). Every mechanical stress on the foot of the mushroom involves the foot-hat juncture, the hats themselves, and the entire system of intracranial suspension and cushioning.

Fig. 2-26: The three-dimensional trampoline or mushroom of the intracranial membrane

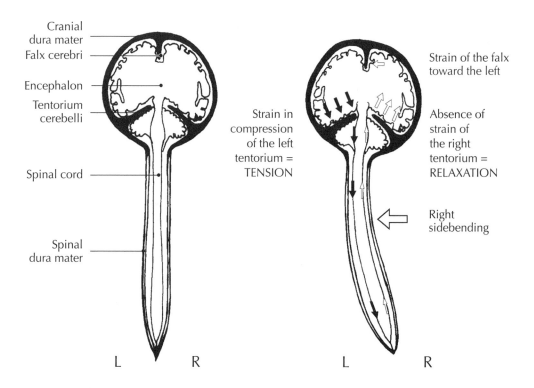

Fig. 2-27: Motion of intracranial membranes during sidebending of the spine
(frontal semischematic section)

belli. The falx, which is contracted by the tentorium, is engaged inferiorly and
posteriorly. Mechanical flexion of the spine reproduces the flexion phase of the
primary respiratory motion.
• by relaxing the PCT and encephalon, spinal extension releases the tentorium
cerebelli. The latter, under the effect of the corrective force of the falx cerebri,
tends to be drawn superiorly and anteriorly. Mechanical extension of the spine
reproduces the conditions of the extension phase of primary respiratory motion.

Sidebending of the spinal cord creates tension in the PCT on the convex side and
relaxation on the concave side. The encephalon is drawn caudad on the convex side and
cephalically on the concave side. During spinal sidebending, the tentorium cerebelli is
preferentially relaxed on the ipsilateral side and is in "high" position. On the side opposite the sidebending, the tentorium is subject to pressure by the encephalon and is in
"low" position *(Fig. 2-27)*.

Effects of horizontal movements on the membranes are more difficult to analyze.
However, we found an interesting study by Breig (1978) on how tic douloureux is triggered by rotation of the head. Since the medulla oblongata is as wide at the foramen
magnum, it can "hug the curve" during rotational head movements. During leftward
rotation of the head, the medulla oblongata and pons deviate laterally toward the left,
which places the root of the right trigeminal nerve under tension *(Fig. 2-28)*. This
phenomenon is associated with difficulty or an obstacle on the trigeminal nerve root
pathway, and explains how leftward rotation of the head can trigger tic douloureux on

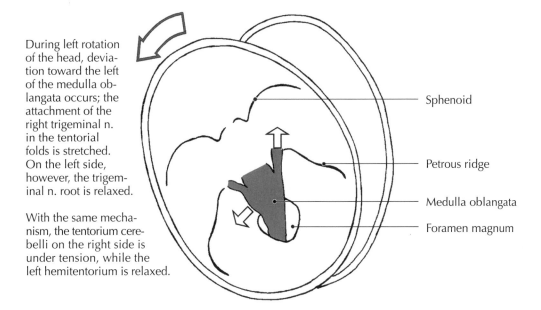

During left rotation of the head, deviation toward the left of the medulla oblangata occurs; the attachment of the right trigeminal n. in the tentorial folds is stretched. On the left side, however, the trigeminal n. root is relaxed.

With the same mechanism, the tentorium cerebelli on the right side is under tension, while the left hemitentorium is relaxed.

Sphenoid

Petrous ridge

Medulla oblangata

Foramen magnum

Fig. 2-28: Tension on the cranial nerves and the tentorium cerebelli during head rotation

the right side.

The important thing to note here is that a leftward rotation produces tension on the right of the medulla oblongata. This tension, which is less marked than that induced by left sidebending, lowers the right side of the tentorium cerebelli and relaxes the left side.

Sidebending or rotation of the spine imposes upon the tentorium cerebelli:

- relaxation and a "high" position on the side of the rotation or sidebending
- tension in the "low" position of the side opposite the movement.

In our opinion, the freedom of this intracranial membranous play is very important in the statics and dynamics of the CNS. Can we imagine cranial mechanics which did not permit lowering of the tentorium cerebelli? What happens to a membrane which loses its slight but necessary elasticity? Small membranous disparities are legion in the sequelae of trauma. The problems they pose for CNS dynamics can be quite disruptive.

To appreciate the interdependence of the two dura mater segments, recall the region of strong osseous adherence in the foramen magnum and the craniospinal hinge area. It is difficult to imagine tissue disequilibrium in one of the two dura mater segments not directly impacting the other. Direct transmission by a fibrous route inside the tissue itself is difficult to imagine because of the strong fibrous ring fixing the dura mater to the osseous parts of the craniospinal hinge.

However, we encounter frequent clinical evidence of a tensile relationship between the two dura matter segments. This relationship appears very complicated and as yet beyond our complete understanding. Our present state of knowledge does not exclude functional complementarity of the two segments *(Fig. 2-29)*.

The mechanical interdependence of the two dura mater segments cannot be based simply on tissue continuity. The adhesions to the cranial bones are important.

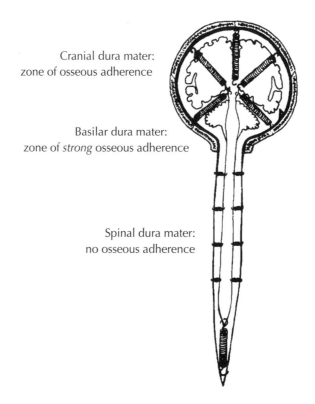

Cranial dura mater:
zone of osseous adherence

Basilar dura mater:
zone of *strong* osseous adherence

Spinal dura mater:
no osseous adherence

Fig. 2-29: Interactions of the two segments of the dura mater

According to our hypothesis, the interdependence also involves the CNS. As if secured and suspended by springs inside each dura mater case, the CNS transmits constraints and disequilibrium from one segment to the next. In this sense, the CNS functions as a craniospinal "mechanical link."

The interdependence seems to occur through CNS statics. There is a mechanical relay through the dentate ligaments and intracranial meningeal structures, which places the cranial and spinal dura mater segments in mechanical communication through interposed nervous tissue.

Pathophysiology

The body is the seat of great tensions of which we are usually unaware. They are compensated for comfortably and easily if the mechanics of the body can adapt freely. For example, we solicit the PCT in many movements and postures of daily life, but it is uncommon that these bother us at all.

After trauma, fundamental mechanical equilibrium mechanisms are disturbed. The tension, which until now had been completely "mute," slowly becomes "expressed." From then on certain movements, activities, or positions become difficult or even painful.

There is often a latency period between the mechanism and appearance of the first symptoms. Additional mechanical stresses over time increase the initial disequilibrium. Movements or mechanical efforts disturb general body harmony and create areas of tissue restriction. Minor tissue or membrane disequilibrium is accentuated. The tissues reinforce each other according to new lines of force which are not physiological (tissue restrictions). The phenomenon of disequilibrium decompensation becomes apparent.

Neuromeningeal disturbances create effects well beyond simple local mechanical disorder. We will describe below several consequences of the disturbance of neuro-meningeal dynamics.

Consequences for the vertebral axis

Spinal functions are usually listed in the following order: stability, mobility, and protection of contents. We believe that the spine is first and foremost an organ of protection, to which the other functions are secondary. All vertebral mechanics are organized for protection of its precious contents.

Study of articular physiology illustrates the many mechanical devices which permit lining up of the axis of the spinal cord or medulla oblongata with transient centers of rotation (e.g., at the level of the atlas and occiput). Every portion of the medulla or cord that is subject to abnormal mechanical stress (e.g., tension, compression, adhesion) can influence mechanical behavior of the surrounding vertebral regions.

When the contents of the spinal column come under stress, there are mechanisms to prevent stress from spreading. Since the spinal dura mater is partially innervated by the sinu-vertebral nerves (also known as the recurrent meningeal nerves), any local or global tissue tension or irritation can serve as a trigger for parietal reflexes. The stimulus is followed by a response of paravertebral muscles which may disturb vertebral mechanics. Reflexes are organized so that posture "avoids" the stressed area, by creating local or regional hypertonia, or sometimes more specific locking of certain mechanical levels.

A thesis study carried out by students in Montreal seems to corroborate this hypothesis. Camirand and Muzzi (1993) demonstrated that osteopathic treatment of the dura mater and its attachments decreases paravertebral muscle tone. This decrease was quantified by electromyelograms and occurred preferentially where there had been peaks of muscular activity preceding treatment, whether or not they were localized. The study included a control group which remained prone for 20 minutes. While a decrease of ~40% in tone was noted in the treatment group, tone in the control group increased by 12%.

According to Louis, any pathological process causing a loss of plasticity of the spinal cord or meninges, or adherence between neuromeningeal structures and the spinal canal walls, can strongly disrupt vertebral motility. This explains arachnoiditis or epiduritis following surgery for a herniated disk. In these cases, lumbar and radicular pain may occur with slight movements of the legs or lumbar spine. Louis stated that maintenance of mobility of the neuromeningeal structures inside the vertebral canal allows stabilization of the natural planes of cleavage between the vertebral contents and container.

These studies confirm the importance of good neuromeningeal dynamics for normal vertebral muscle tone.

We believe that the vertebral axis reacts either globally or segmentally to nociceptive information from the viscera of the trunk. We have seen many cases of vertebral pain secondary to irritations or loss of mobility in the digestive viscera.

Even though the vertebral container may "respect" its neurological contents, it may also behave dysfunctionally because of them. Cervical stiffness (sometimes even stiffness of the entire spine) during meningitis is a good illustration. The stiffness demonstrates the intensity of the reflex phenomenon when neuromeningeal contents are irritated.

This principle helps us better understand certain postmanipulative pain reactions. In our experience, vertebral manipulation is rarely indicated as a first step. Simple treatment of the cerebrospinal axis and its envelopes permits easy, completely pain-free manipulation, without pressure and without danger.

Neuromeningeal restrictions of the vertebral column are a frequent cause of recurring pain. We all have patients who return again and again with the same complaint and the same restrictions, even though they should have been cured by our manipulations. Often, following trauma, myotensive or structural vertebral articular techniques are indicated only after release of the duromedullary axis.

Consequences for the intervertebral disks

The disks dehydrate during the day as a result of the load applied to them. During the night, because gravitational stress is removed in the recumbent position, they become rehydrated and their mechanical capacities are renewed by the morning. This nocturnal rehydration requires phases of deep and rapid eye movement sleep to obtain muscular relaxation. We believe that complete freedom of the spinal dura mater is also indispensable. In cases of tension, adherence, or meningeal fibrosis, the dura mater can prevent normal intervertebral decompression and disrupt nocturnal rehydration of the disk. Over the long term, certain aspects of disk degeneration may be enhanced by this mechanism.

Consequences for the autonomic system

The upper part of the PCT is anatomically continuous with the diencephalon, and the mechanical endpoint of the PCT corresponds to the hypothalamus and thalamus. The thalamus contains many autonomic centers and may be considered, physiologically, to govern autonomic functions.

Permanent stress by traction on the PCT or restriction of the tentorium cerebelli can cause chronic autonomic stimulation. We believe that trauma is often the cause of autonomic dystonia. There is often a latency period between the traumatic event and the appearance of the first pathological signs, so that the patient is not aware of the cause-effect relationship.

Patients who present with severe autonomic dystonia have responses which are disproportionate relative to injury or daily stress. These include behavioral problems, mood swings, and emotional problems.

Clinical and experimental studies of brain lesions confirm the importance of the brainstem in mechanisms involving awareness and vigilance. Several structures of the upper PCT play a primary role in the wake-sleep mechanisms. On one hand:

- the *reticular formation* which extends throughout the top of the brainstem
- the *locus ceruleus* situated at the upper part of the brainstem, near the lateral wall of the fourth ventricle.

The more these regions are stimulated at the neuronal level, the more they act together to maintain the subject in a state of awareness. Anatomically, they are in a position of intense mechanical stress during daily activities. Mechanical stimulation probably occurs on a physiological as well as neuronal level.

On the other hand:

- the *thalamus* and *hypothalamus* play a role in maintaining awareness. A nucleus in the posterior hypothalamus promotes waking and an adjacent nucleus in the anterior hypothalamus promotes sleep.

Sleep is frequently decreased (hyposomnia or insomnia) or increased (hyper-somnia) following trauma. These problems can be related to disrupted mechanics of the PCT, and should not be hastily labeled as signs of depression or post-traumatic stress disorder.

Neuroendocrinological consequences

For mechanical reasons as above, certain neuroendocrine dysfunctions may be related to trauma. The pituitary is located under the hypothalamus and may be disturbed by permanent mechanical stimulation of the PCT. Also, pituitary hormones are diverted to the intercavernous sinus, whose walls are comprised of lateral extensions of tentorium cerebelli insertions. Abnormal tension from the tentorium can induce local circulatory disturbances which do not disrupt secretion, but rather its access to the general circulation.

Feedback regulation of pituitary secretion occurs by inhibition of the factors triggering the secretion. The logistical support for this regulation is circulatory, and the fragile hormonal balance may change if the vascular beds are disturbed.

Since the major part of the intracranial venous system is incorporated in the edges of the dura mater, any abnormal tension on the dura mater or PCT can disturb local blood flow.

Once hormonal balance has been disrupted, it is difficult for normal endocrine physiology to be reestablished. Functional signs appear which are intermittent at first, but become more pronounced over time. Neuroendocrine dysfunction can have serious medium- or long-term homeostatic consequences, including the following:

- reproduction:
  - dysmenorrhea
  - amenorrhea
  - reduced libido

- metabolism:
  - weight gain
  - bulimia, cravings
  - loss of appetite
  - diffuse digestive problems

- basal tone of autonomic and somatic systems:
  - cold intolerance
  - sleep disturbances
  - depressed state
  - neurasthenia, with difficulties of attention and memorization
  - problems performing activities of daily living.

Intracavity and Visceral Lesions

We described the differences in luminal pressures previously (Barral & Mercier, 1988). The negative pressure of the thorax greatly decreases the effective weight of various organs. It also permits blood and lymph circulation with minimal energy expenditure and provides the basis of the turgor effect.

Remember the example of the liver whose average weight of 1.5kg is transformed to an effective weight of 300-400g by thoracodiaphragmatic attraction. This phenomenon can occur only if the tissues involved maintain normal tone, extensibility, and elasticity, and effectively transmit differences in pressure.

Thorax

In experiments with pigs, the French National Institute for Research on Transportation and Safety (INRETS) demonstrated that resistance of the thorax to impact cannot be attributed solely to the thoracic cage (Verriest, 1986). They showed that *during trauma, resistance to thoracic compression is also based on inertia and viscosity of the intrathoracic viscera.* The greater the speed of compression, the more significant this phenomenon. For this reason, the severity of visceral injury is not proportional to number of rib fractures, as long as the latter do not perforate the pleura or peritoneum (Anselmet, 1985).

In many cases of significant trauma, the organs help protect the thoracic cage. Visceral manipulations following trauma are therefore particularly important. The thoracic cage receives strong pressure which is transmitted to the organs and retransmitted. Restrictions of ligaments of organ attachment, particularly the cervicopleural and sternomediastinal ligaments, are very important in diagnosis and treatment.

Abdomen

The abdomen is not surrounded by a bony cage like the thorax. It is protected only partially by the lesser pelvis and vertebral column. The organs are viscoelastic masses like the brain. They are suspended from the diaphragm, or more rarely by ligaments from bones. These ligaments have very sensitive mechanoreceptors.

Shock waves are focused on the hardest organs (liver, spleen, kidneys). The organs in turn abnormally stress their support ligaments which then either strengthen, excite, or (more rarely) destroy their mechanoreceptors. The receptors send signals causing local, regional, or central responses such as pain, spasm, and organ restriction. Visceral mobility and motility are compromised, the mechanoreceptors no longer transmit correct information relative to intracavity pressure, and the turgor effect is decreased. Effective weight of the organ increases and "drags down" the diaphragm and the lymphovenous circulation.

Most lesions occur where ligamentous stresses are significant. Following severe trauma, lesions are more common on the left side near the spleen and left kidney. The frequency of splenic fracture demonstrates the fragility of this organ, and the concentration of forces from collision on the left side. The mediastinum and pericardium disperse the forces of collision laterally in order to protect the heart. These forces are often directed obliquely downward and to the left in the direction of the spleen and left kidney. A plausible biomechanical explanation for the concentration of mechanical lesions on the left is described in Chapter 5.

Chapter Three:
A Tissular Approach to Trauma

Table of Contents

A Tissular Approach to Trauma

Reactivity of Tissue to Impact

In analyses of the consequences of trauma, it is often assumed that tissues are isotropic (having identical physical properties in all directions), homogeneous, and transmit shock from collision in a straight line. In reality, living tissues react to impact in different ways. Consider the brain. Its tissues are quite heterogeneous: white matter, gray matter, ventricles, cerebrospinal fluid, hard and soft meninges, neurons. Each of these tissues transmits and assimilates shock waves in different ways. They are definitely not equal from a vibrational point of view!

Note: Parenchymatous and vascular changes occur at the junction of structures with different moments of inertia.

In addition to the complex mechanical factors involved, biological, chemical, hormonal, and psychological reactions also come into play following lesions. The acute stage of concussion, for example, is characterized by an abnormality of perfusion in the frontotemporal region due to movement of intracerebral fluids, in addition to neurochemical phenomena (Maideu, 1991).

Tolerance to impact

Tissues faced with impact are capable of adaptation and compensation. But successful adaptation is dependent upon the force and direction of impact. "Objective" mechanicophysical data have been taken from dummies and inert bodies (anesthetized or dead). These studies are interesting but must be interpreted with caution.

During trauma the large amount of cervical mobility helps compensate for the force of collision exerted on the skull. This mobility reduces the effect of the forces at the osseous level, while increasing it in the soft tissues (brain, meninges, muscles, ligaments). At the moment of impact the skull is significantly deformed for about 50 milliseconds, causing direct contusion of the brain and underlying soft tissues.

Cerebral lesions

Lesions to the brain following impact are caused primarily by shear stress. Three important mechanical factors are:

- post-traumatic intracranial pressure gradients
- skull deformation upon impact
- movements of the cerebral mass in the skull.

Contusions

Contusions are a type of microhemorrhage or petechial hemorrhage occurring at the point of impact or opposite to it. They create significant edema preventing normal brain functioning, leading to abnormal cerebral electrical conduction.

Neuronal lesions

Stresses due to angular acceleration often cause parenchymatous lesions of the nervous system. They directly affect the axons of the longitudinal tracts forming the white matter.

- A slight acceleration or deceleration suspends axonal flux and causes a brief cerebral coma.
- Intense and sustained acceleration or deceleration stretches and breaks millions of axons, causing a prolonged coma.
- In violent trauma, the shock wave can completely destroy neurons. The prognosis depends upon the quality and quantity of neurons destroyed.

Concept of osseous intracavity stress

Shearing stress affects primarily the intracavity irregularities related either to the bones or disks. In the skull, irregularities are found at the anterior part of the skull base, orbital surface of frontal lobes, and temporal region. In the spine, shearing stress leads to problems such as uncarthrosis (disease of the uncinate processes of C3 to T1), osteophytes (bony excrescence), disk arthrosis, discopathy, and stenosis.

Note: Craniospinal intracavity volume and pressure must remain constant for normal CNS functioning. Variation in these two components due to an abnormal bony or disk obstacle has pathological effects which may appear far from the obstacle itself. For example, consider a patient who suffers cervical whiplash. If he has uncarthrosis at the level of C6, the forces of collision are focused here. If, in addition, he has an intracanal L4/L5 discopathy, intracanal pressure is even greater and forces of collision are even more destructive at the level of C6. Increase and concentration of intracanal pressure causes a restriction, which is aggravated by the lack of general compensation of the L5/S1 disk arthrosis.

The forces of collision are always focused at the point of maximal intracanal stress. A fall on the coccyx sometimes creates a restriction of cervical vertebrae if the latter are fixed or arthrosed.

Proprioceptive "disinformation"

During trauma, mechanoreceptors are subjected to rough treatment. In addition

RE ACTIVITY OF TISSUE TO IMPACT

to the osteoarticular system, mechanoreceptors are found in the visceral and perhaps craniosacral systems.

They react to strong mechanical force by "disinforming" local, regional, or central nerve centers. They either underestimate or overestimate the mechanical stimuli received. This proprioceptive "disinformation" causes inappropriate muscular reactions which endanger the patient's general equilibrium, and lead to leg or ankle sprains due to poor contraction or muscular coordination.

Vascular lesions

Of mechanical origin

At the cerebral and cerebellar level, vascular lesions are primarily venous. The superior veins have thin walls, which are sensitive to mechanical lesions affecting the internal table of the bone and the dura mater. Remember that the dura mater adheres to bone except where it surrounds venous tissues.

Cranial trauma causes osseous deformation, detaching the dura mater from the bone. In general, lesions are from direct impact and not from a projected impact from the opposite side. Venous or arterial dissections cause extradural hematoma.

Extradural or subdural hematomas are common at the frontal level, due to rupture of the median meningeal artery or dural venous sinuses. Vascular lesions are frequently caused by acceleration or deceleration, with a temporal delay between the movement undergone by the head and that disturbing the brain.

Of reflex origin

Mechanical attack of certain nerves or nerve centers (particularly in the bulbar area) can cause lasting vasoconstriction in certain regions of the brain, cerebellum, or even spinal cord.

We have observed lasting neurological injuries such as paresthesias which seem to have no topographical explanation. They can sometimes be explained by vasoconstriction of the spinal artery or major anterior radicular arteries causing poor circulation to the spinal cord.

Hormonal-chemical reactions

When parenchymatous areas are affected either directly or indirectly by trauma, many complex biochemical reactions occur which can lead to circulatory problems and edema. Following trauma, neurotransmitters are very active, leading to hypersecretion of catecholamines, kinins, arachidonic acid, serotonin, histamine, and perhaps other as yet undiscovered substances. These substances cause invasion of extracellular spaces by protein macromolecules and water, leading to edema, which compresses tissues such as the white matter.

Many post-traumatic syndromes and resulting neurasthenia are not purely psychogenic in origin. It is not surprising that such trauma patients feel unwell because of the increase in neurotransmitter secretion. Female patients may experience amenorrhea (or more rarely, polymenorrhea) after trauma. We certainly do not deny the existence of psychological causes, but think that mechanical problems also affect function of the pituitary gland and hypothalamus.

Topographical effects

During trauma, the forces of collision enter the body at the area of impact. The shock wave is then propagated through the body as a function of tissue density. The wave is not linear, and numerous examples demonstrate that it is transmitted in apparently illogical directions. Listening is an indispensable part of osteopathic assessment, as it often picks up shock wave pathways that cannot be found using any conventional form of imaging technology.

One injury can cause several shock waves, as when a pebble is thrown into the water, with different shock waves having different pathways. Sacrococcygeal trauma may cause only cervical or cranial restrictions, or it may lead to localized problems.

Entry and exit of the energy of collision

From the point of impact, the shock waves can:

- be concentrated rapidly on a precise region, causing a major lesion such as a fracture or tear
- traverse a long distance in the body, slowly losing momentum, until they disappear. Many lesions occur, but they are not serious.
- traverse a long distance with ever increasing pressure against a solid element at the end of the path, causing a major lesion
- much more rarely, traverse the body without causing any harm. We can recall patients who suffered no serious damage after a fall from a high elevation or a major car or train accident.

Effect in time

Immediate

After trauma, the body tends to "favor" the most intense pain. The most seriously affected region is not always the one that gives the most nociceptive information. A patient may consult about a pain which has no obvious pathological basis; the body is fooled by the immediate symptoms.

We had a patient who suffered a very painful fracture of the ankle bone following a motorcycle accident and was found to have a hemopneumothorax several months later. This pneumothorax could have had severe consequences. It was only after the fracture healed that the pleuropulmonary symptoms developed.

Mediator effects

Even if an injury has only one region of impact it may create lesions far from the trauma and for a long time after its occurrence. The damaged parts may be found all along the pathway of the shock wave. The latter may even have a circular trajectory in the skull. As a cure is achieved for one problem, other lesions appear, which are sometimes very hard to explain.

Reactivity of patients to trauma

All people react differently to trauma, depending on genetic predisposition, tissue properties, cumulative effects, previous injuries, and individual degrees of central and psychological reactivity. Some patients present significant ecchymoses from trivial impact. Some hypersensitive patients suffer greatly from trauma which would not even be noticed by less sensitive individuals.

In view of this wide range of individual reactivity, we must respect the patient's symptoms without making judgments or moralizing, and especially without making comparisons. We should be more understanding than a practitioner who, after hearing the litany of a patient's complaints, tells a "similar" story of his own, presenting himself as an example of someone who "reacts well." A slight case of whiplash in a patient with degenerative disease of the cervical spine can be much more painful and pathogenic than a similar case in a patient with a healthy spine.

Psychological reactions

The tissues preserve the memory of a trauma. Our instinct for self-preservation causes us to be afraid when we are in real or imagined danger. Injury is always accompanied by a conscious and unconscious psychological reaction.

A slowly-developing dangerous situation is recorded in the conscious memory. When the danger and the force of collision from a traumatic impact occur very suddenly, without time for conscious awareness, they are perceived and stored in the unconscious. Remember that a collision event can occur within fifty milliseconds, much too fast for conscious perception.

Psychological memory of trauma

The danger, force of collision, reactive lesions, and pain sensations combine to create negative psychological information. This information triggers immediate reactions such as fear, panic, syncope, and somatization. But it is also relayed to and stored in various memory centers of the brain and other parts of the CNS or body, such as the nerve plexus.

The psychological memory of trauma becomes an integral part of the individual's life. When another accident occurs, the psychological effects may be out of proportion to the severity of the accident, because of a cumulative effect.

Cumulative effects

Traumatic impact always awakens the memory of another trauma. Seemingly minor injuries can therefore have devastating effects on the pyschological equilibrium of an individual. We must abstain from judging individual reactions to trauma by our own standards.

We believe that at the tissue level there are physical and psychological memories associated with past traumatic or emotional events. It is impossible to obtain rigorous proof of this concept, but clinical experience bears it out every day. Tissue memory is not only physical. In our practice, this is frequently illustrated by post-manipulation reactions disproportionate to the corrective context. We believe that psychological memories may reside in various body tissues, and that these memories are capable of stimulating certain cortical centers.

Lesion Activity

Release vs. accumulation of the energy of collision

When the force of collision is concentrated in one direction and on one point (a very hypothetical situation), a tissue tear or fracture will result. In the skull, this is sometimes preferable to an internal tissue lesion, since the force of collision disperses and disappears by expressing itself in the fracture. But what happens if the force is not expressed in this way?

According to the concept of the accumulation of energy, any body tissue can retain a part of the force of collision which has not been expressed in a structural lesion. This concept explains the frequent cases in which symptoms disappear or then recur months or even years after the traumatic event. The energy of collision is often stored in an asymptomatic, "silent" manner.

The body retains the memory of trauma. Even an asymptomatic fall on the behind at five years of age becomes part of a patient's "inheritance."

Compensation-adaptation

Every tissue lesion, whether producing symptoms or not, is stored by the body. A complex system of compensation and adaptation helps prevent pain and functional disability.

As a simple example, a knee sprain may be compensated for by the underlying osteoarticular system. However, the sprain leaves its imprint in not only the ligamentous capsule and synovial fibers, but also the spinal and central proprioceptive centers. A second sprain, even if less severe, will create its own lesions, awaken old ones, and possibly have serious consequences. Mechanisms by which a small impact can cause serious problems include:

- tissue memory
- decrease in adaptation-compensation capacity
- central cord facilitation.

Lesion Pathophysiology and Symptoms

Muscles

Muscle fibers are 10 to 100mm wide and up to 15cm long. Seen under a microscope, they form longitudinal striations interrupted by transverse striations. The structural unit of muscle is called the sarcomere.

Pathomechanics

In the event of trauma, muscle structure may change and some fibers may break as they exceed the threshold of elasticity and distention. In addition, the fiber will atrophy if its blood supply or innervation is compromised by trauma.

Direct muscle trauma

The viscoelastic qualities of muscle help it tolerate direct trauma reasonably well. However, it can be damaged and superficially or deeply crushed to various degrees.

- Simple contusion is the least serious lesion. It is a rupture of several muscle fibers, with formation of a small hematoma which infiltrates the muscle body, and sometimes a tear of the aponeurosis.
- Crushing injury of the muscle body may or may not involve breaking of the skin. It adds a large hematoma to an extensive lesion of muscle fibers.

INDIRECT MUSCLE TRAUMA

Indirect muscle lesions occur during sports-related trauma, or domestic or automobile accidents. The lesion is always closed, and involves rupture of muscle fibers and formation of hematomas of various sizes.

- *Elongation* causes sharp pain and discrete edema related to a lesion of several muscle fibers. Elongation is not serious, but rather serves as a signal for general disturbance, violent movement, or muscle fatigue.
- *Pulled muscles* occur mainly in athletes, often during relaxation movements in tennis, sprinting, basketball, volleyball, and other sports. A pulled muscle is accompanied by pain, slight limitation of movement, and often a sensation of dry clicking. It corresponds to the rupture of several muscle fibers.
- *Tear (rupture)* results from extensive strain, and may involve one or several muscle tracts. The tear is perpendicular to the fiber direction, and usually situated in the middle of the muscle fiber. A large hematoma is formed, but aponeurotic integrity causes it to remain inside the muscle and not diffuse to surrounding tissues.

MUSCLE DEGENERATION OF TRAUMATIC ORIGIN

Muscle degeneration can result from direct trauma, or from injury to the muscle's blood supply or innervation.

- *Muscular necrosis* of vascular origin is an aseptic myosis which depends upon the extent of the lesion.
- *Degeneration* of nerve origin leads to muscle atrophy.

Hypothesis on sarcomere deformation

We believe that trauma is followed by deformation of the sarcomeres in the longitudinal and, more rarely, transverse direction. A sarcomere's actin and myosin filaments are arranged to fit together, and the sliding of filaments causes the muscle to shorten. Deformation of the sarcomeres may prevent this sliding, and cause abnormal stimuli leading to abnormal muscle tension. Such deformations may slightly change the axis of muscular contraction and distort the mobility and motility of a part of the body.

Each muscle fiber is enclosed by a connective tissue sheath, the sarcolemma, which is involved in mechanical disruption of muscle function if its extensibility is impaired.

REGIONS OF HYPODENSITY AND HYPERDENSITY

A mechanical lesion acts on local vasomotor activity through its effect on the nervous system. Individual muscle cells experience hypocirculation (or more rarely, hypercirculation). Muscle regions of lower density, which are difficult to recognize by most forms of palpation, may be detected with listening. Regions of hyperdensity may be formed at the beginning of trauma, in edema and fluid stasis, as well as some scarring processes.

ELECTROMAGNETIC FIELD OF LESIONS

An intriguing question is why certain tendinous and fascial lesions cause a pathological process years later. These processes are identified by techniques of osteopathic diagnosis which are rarely demonstrable by "objective" techniques.

Why are apparently healthy tissues capable of disorganizing a postural scheme? Clinical experience demonstrates that all trauma leaves an imprint upon bodily tissues which is only revealed by CT scan, MRI, or ultrasound in cases of extreme deterioration. At the present time, only thermal scans objectively demonstrate that the electromagnetic field surrounding damaged regions is different from that of neighboring regions.

Skeletal tissues

Because it is practically always involved in trauma, skeletal tissue has been the subject of countless studies. Here, we will simply highlight a few points essential for understanding the consequences of trauma on skeletal tissues.

The skeleton should be viewed as a composite tissue fulfilling numerous functions. There are two types of skeletal tissue:

- cartilaginous: resistant but elastic tissue. The fetal skeleton is primarily cartilaginous, while the adult skeleton contains only a small proportion of this material.
- osseous: solid, hard, inflexible material. Bones are often thought of inaccurately as inert materials, but are in fact very much "alive." They are capable of adaptation, regeneration, and healing like the majority of bodily tissues, and may be the site of tumors, infections, or fractures.

A mechanical imperative of all soft body tissues is "dampening." Every mechanical system of the human body has dampening properties, which are stressed by trauma. The skeletal tissues, despite their hardness, share this property.

Bone and periosteum

Bone is an organ with multiple functions:

- a mechanical organ which provides support, mobility, and protection
- participates actively in phosphate calcium metabolism
- contributes to maintenance of blood calcium level, an important constant of the internal environment
- a hematopoietic organ which contains the bone marrow, the major supplier of blood cells and other elements.

Bone tissue

Bone tissue is composed of a frame of collagen and mineral salts, in which the bone cells (osteocytes) are distributed. The composition of the osseous substance changes from birth to old age, and the ratio of collagen to mineral salts also varies, with the mineral salts tending to predominate over time.

Mature bone, referred to as a "biphasic" material, is composed of 70% inorganic constituents (mainly phosphate and calcium) and 30% organic materials (mostly collagen). Bone tissue is essentially a calcium impregnation of an organic matrix with the composition of connective tissue.

Bone tissue never comes into direct contact with the other tissues. Its articular surfaces are covered by hyaline cartilage and its nonarticular parts by periosteum, a richly innervated and vascularized fibrous membrane. Internally, the bone is isolated from the marrow by the endosteal layer.

Bone tissue has two subtypes.

Compact bone:

- constitutes the peripheral layer of the diaphysis of the long bones, short bones, and flat bones
- is made up of a multitude of cylinders (osteons) characterized by concentric osseous lamellae, grouped around a central haversian canal.

Spongy bone:

- fills the epiphyses and metaphyses of the long bones, and the center of the short bones and flat bones. In the calvaria, it forms the diploe, or spongy tissue between the inner and outer tables.
- comprised of osseous lamellae arranged in anastomized and interleaved spans, "bathed" by red or yellow bone marrow. The direction of the osseous trabeculations determines the lines of force by which sprains occur within the osseous tissue. This architectural factor is important for osseous resistance, allowing for some dampening under the cartilaginous articular surfaces.

Points of ossification

Ossification begins at the end of the embryonic period, as the cartilaginous or membranous matrix is progressively replaced by bone tissue.

There are two types of ossification:

- from connective tissue, or ossification of the membrane
- from cartilaginous tissue, or chondral ossification.

Bone formation proceeds in two stages: appearance of a point of primary ossification, and then one or several points of secondary ossification.

Primary points of ossification appear during the intrauterine period. They are located at the diaphysis or in the center of bones, at the invasion of the primary vascular bud. Ossification then proceeds in the direction of the epiphyses or the periphery.

Secondary points of ossification appear in the epiphyses or at the periphery of bones during the postnatal period, sometimes just before birth. The region where the points of ossification are fused together constitute the *epiphyseal line.*

Points of ossification appear and are fused at different ages, permitting evaluation of growth stage. Compared to an adult, a child has a larger number of osseous parts which, separated by cartilage growth disks, permit better tolerance to impact during childhood. Growth and osseous mineralization progressively render this osteocartilaginous skeleton denser, and it gradually loses its youthful elasticity.

Mechanical properties of bone tissue

The fundamental mechanical properties of living bone are *elasticity* and *resistance*; although these seem to be contradictory, they grant the bone tissue its unique character. Spongy tissue has less physical resistance than compact tissue, and is more easily crushed or penetrated (meshed epiphyseal fracture).

Bone is an anisotropic material which is 1.5 to 2 times more resistant in compression than in traction. This is borne out by the variability of its modulus (coefficient) of elasticity. Young's modulus of elasticity for a long bone decreases from the endosteal layer to the periosteum, which permits harmonious distribution of sprains in the cortical bone.

Young's modulus of elasticity for a bone takes into consideration age, sex, type of bone, and type of force applied. Spongy bone has a modulus roughly a third that of cortical bone. It is only slightly resistant to the strains of torsion and radial compression.

Bone is a viscoelastic material. Under a load, a bone is progressively deformed for 55 days, at which time deformation reaches 153% of that which occurs in two minutes. In other words, bone has greater resistance to rapid than slow deformation.

Clinical application

Bone grows well only when subject to mechanical stress. When these stresses occur outside their normal axis and are repeatedly poorly damped, the spans and osteons are deformed, leading to deformation. Increasing the force of compression on a bone leads to hypertrophy. If forces are too strong, osseous lysis occurs. When stress on a bone is decreased (as when confined to bed, in space, or paralyzed), osteoporosis and fragile tissue result.

Mechanical pathology of the tissue

The elastic properties of bone tissues give them the ability to dampen impact. Above an upper load limit in violent trauma, the reversibility of normally elastic deformation ceases. This excessive deformation is expressed in various degrees of rupture of the bony tissue.

CONCEPT OF FRACTURE

Borgi and Plas (1982) proposed an interesting definition of fracture: "Fracture is a *dissolution of continuity* in the bone tissue, separating the bone into two or more fragments. Its cause is most often violent trauma (provoked fracture) but also may be a harmless gesture (spontaneous fracture). Functionally, fracture is disorganization of the musculoskeletal system by abolition of the transmission of a load . . ." Thus, a fracture is defined by its location, type, features, and possible displacement.

MECHANISM OF FRACTURE

The mechanism of fracture can be direct or indirect. Direct fracture occurs as a result of collision between the bone and an external object. The cause is most often violence and contusion or crushing of the skin. When the mechanism is indirect, the fracture occurs at a distance from the point of impact. There are four categories of indirect fracture: those due to compression, traction, torsion, and flexion.

Fractures caused by compression and by traction

Fractures due to compression cause compacting or indentation, and those caused by traction are the result of tearing. The direction of the traumatic force applied to the bone is identical in both cases; only the direction changes.

Fractures of the calcaneus and of the vertebral body are typically due to compression. They cause compacting through crushing of the spongy bone. Fractures of the coronoid process of the ulna and of the greater tubercle of the humerus occur through an indirect traction mechanism, due to violent stress of tendinous-muscular origin.

Fractures caused by torsion and by flexion

Torsion fractures result from a coupling of forces causing circular action on the bone. These fractures are spiral. This is the case with fractures that occur while skiing, when bodily rotation is attempted with the ankle fixed. The tibia separates into two fragments.

Flexion fractures can be compared to flexing of a beam. They are characterized by forces of compression and traction. Stresses from compression are localized on the concave side and those from traction on the convex side. This is true of fractures of the neck of the femur, for example.

Fatigue-induced fractures

These are osseous lesions which occur after a series of repetitive but relatively gentle traumas. They are frequently experienced by athletes and military personnel, especially on the neck of the femur and the bones of the feet.

SEVERITY OF FRACTURES

Independent of mechanism, the severity of a fracture is always tied to the risk of damaging some life-sustaining tissues of the body. In fact, loss of mechanical qualities by a bony segment is not necessarily serious. It is the risk of hemorrhage, or vascular or neurological lesion, that defines a serious fracture.

Functional approach

THE ROLE OF THE PERIOSTIUM

Unlike bone, the periostium is richly innervated and vascularized. Its external fibrous layer joins the fibers of insertion of tendons, fasciae, and muscles. Any myofascial injury has repercussions on the periostium and bone, and is capable of deforming them.

Following trauma, even without fracture, deformations of skeletal structures occur over time. They are due to:

- hypovascularization of connective and osseous tissues
- dysfunction of chondrocytes and osteocytes
- demineralization and injury of the interstitial cartilaginous substance
- poor dampening of mechanical stresses.

Hyaline cartilage contains numerous collagen and elastic fibers in its ground substance. From the moment the viscoelasticity of the fascia attached to the periostium is disturbed, abnormal tension is capable of deforming the periostium and bone. This deformation, occuring over a period of years, reveals the poor underlying transmission of the mechanical forces received by the connective and bony tissues.

The periosteum contains mechanoreceptors connected to the sympathetic inner-vation of muscles, tendons, and fascia. These mechanoreceptors are also vasomotor, and exert an effect on vasomotor activity of the periosteal arteries.

Any slowing of arterial flow influences the venous-lymphatic system as well as cellular density. In the event of cellular hypodensity, periosteal viscoelasticity is less effective, and the mechanical injury receives less dampening and compensation.

Cartilage

Articular cartilage is a connective tissue which lacks blood or lymph vessels and nerves, and covers the articular edges of the bones. Its lack of vascularization makes it dependent upon synovial fluid and subchondral bone for nutrition. Articular cartilage is an excellent illustration of the adaptation of biological tissue to function:

- it guarantees coherent distribution of stress on the osseous surfaces
- participates in articular sliding movements with a low friction coefficient
- helps dampen impact during daily activities and trauma.

Composition and mechanical properties

Cartilage constitutes an articular contact interface from 2-4mm thick with a smooth, pearly white surface. Composed of 75% water, with a density of $1.3g/cm^3$, it has a modulus of elasticity of $11.1 \times 106N/m^2$, or 1,000 times less that of water. This explains its ability to undergo deformation without rupturing.

Cartilage is very elastic, but is anisotropic like bone tissue. Its response varies depending upon the type of stress applied. Its resistance to compression depends upon its concentration of water and proteoglycans, while its resistance to traction depends upon the collagen fibers. A mechanical model for cartilage is a hydrophilic gel with tightly binding collagen fibers.

Cartilage is lubricated by synovial fluid, which has a resistance of 10 to 100kg-cm^2. Its lubricating capacity is excellent since its coefficient of friction is on the order of 10 to 4 (0.0001 to 0.0032)—lower than that of a skate on ice. Manufacturers of industrial lubricants allow coefficients of friction of approximately 10 to 2 (0.01).

Mechanical pathology of cartilage

The elasticity of cartilage makes it highly compressible and extensible. Repeated stresses lead to formation of cracks and lines on the surface. Articular wounds, fractures, and dislocation can damage cartilage, but it is rarely damaged from simple contusion.

Degenerative lesions of cartilage can occur as a result of even slight trauma. In certain conditions, lesions tend to progress to the deep layers and may resemble arthrotic lesions by the sixth month.

Pathological trauma to the articular cartilage

EPIDEMIOLOGY

Violent trauma can fracture the epiphyses, injuring the spongy bone and articular cartilage. Any articular injury can cause a chondral or osteochondral fracture, which is often difficult to diagnose, and may not be discovered until much later. Indirect traumas seem to pose the greatest danger to cartilaginous tissue.

Fractures in adults occur at the area of weakness at the border of the calcified and hyaline layers of the articular cartilage, which releases a purely cartilaginous fragment. Since children and adolescents have no calcified cartilage, a rupture bypasses the subchondral bone, releasing an osteocartilaginous fragment. The fragment may become a "foreign body," a free, mobile agent, and source of problems or restriction, whose diagnosis reveals the articular injury. In a young child, certain epiphyseal fractures traverse the nucleus of ossification without touching the growth plaque. X-rays reveal a fragmentary nucleus of ossification.

Direct contusions compress the cartilage and subchondral bone, which breaks or is deformed into a cup-like shape. These contusions are probably the cause of certain cases of osteochondrosis or necrosis. Too much capsular-ligamentous or tendinous traction can cause an osteocartilaginous tear, which may be quite large. The area scars to varying degrees. Actual healing, with reconstruction of the hyaline cartilage, occurs rarely. More often, scarring creates fibrocartilage whose long-term resistance is unpredictable.

ARCHITECTURE OF JOINTS

A slight digression into articular geometry is in order. Industrially, if one wanted to make two perfect spheres, one inside the other, it would be necessary to machine them to very low tolerance. They would have to be positioned with extreme precision, so that all points are equidistant from one another. If the two surfaces were not completely congruent, considerable force would be focused on the points of contact and cause significant deformation.

Nature resolves this type of problem in mammalian joints by interposing a force-absorbing material—cartilage—between the two surfaces. The cartilage is covered by synovia, which further equalize the stresses. Nonetheless, surface irregularities within the joint which arise following trauma will still cause stress at certain points of articulation. Normal activity of peri-articular muscles (which act as articular "locks") contributes to the loads and stresses on the joints.

In summary, disturbances of the epiphyseal architecture or regularity of the cartilage have an adverse effect on joints, resulting in premature pain and arthrosis. The reaction of the cartilage to weak but repetitive trauma is not always adaptation. Degeneration of cartilage begins in the second decade of life, even in healthy individuals.

The evolution of cartilaginous lesions in response to regular trauma occurs in progressive phases. At first, the lesions are reversible. Arthritic degeneration of the cartilage involves an initial stage of chondritis.

Pathophysiology

Chondritis is the primary response of cartilage to trauma. The thickness and water content of the cartilage markedly increase. This stage, called *edematous chondritis*, is reversible.

The next stage, in which the regularity of the surface is disturbed by persistent edema, is partially reversible, and is called *ulcerative chondritis*. If not treated, this leads to chronic ulcerative chondritis, which is irreversible, and includes outgrowths on the edges of the articular surface.

Post-traumatic arthrosis has many manifestations. The range of articular mobility is very narrow and restricted by the ligaments. Abnormality of mobility can cause cartilaginous lesions through alteration of the speed, distribution, or direction of stresses.

Two phenomena determine development of arthrosis:

- gradual degeneration of the cartilage, causing articular incongruence, which modifies the forces of compression and traction exerted on the cartilage
- rapid degeneration of cartilage during severe contusions or crushing. A simple contusion of cartilage can lead to almost immediate necrosis of the chondrocytes, causing degeneration (Trias, 1961).

During crushing or cutting of the articular cartilage, the chondrocytes die from the following causes:

- loss of proteoglycans
- fissure formation
- erosion
- eburnation (a disorganization and fragmentation of the superficial layer of cartilage, and extension of degeneration to deeper layers).

Subchondral spongy bone tissue plays a major role in dampening cartilaginous pressure. Epiphyseal bone that is too dense can cause pressure overload on cartilage. Osteopathic techniques which restore malleability to the bone tissue may be helpful in this case, and for some types of arthrosis.

Trauma to the growth cartilage

Trauma to a growing skeleton is frequent, varied in type and location, yet rapidly cured.

Skeletal tissue in a young subject has great dampening capacity. Likewise, falls during infancy or adolescence are generally much better tolerated than in adulthood. This is due to the constitution of the bony segments themselves, which are comprised of osseous tissue nuclei separated by bands of cartilaginous tissue which are responsible for skeletal growth. This arrangement results in greater elasticity of the skeleton and better tolerance of impact. However, even though traumas of childhood are less likely to cause fractures, they are not always innocuous.

The greatest danger is destruction of the growth cartilage, by alteration of the germinal layer leading to epiphysiodesis (premature union of the epiphysis with the diaphysis). Partial epiphysiodesis causes axial deviation of the limb, while total epiphysiodesis causes shortening of the bone and the affected limb.

There are many types of joint injury which involve separation or detachment of cartilage. *However, lesions to growth cartilage are the most dangerous. Also, being invisible on x-ray, they are difficult to diagnose.*

Epiphysiodesis is most well known in relation to limb trauma, but can also occur in the axial skeleton. Childhood trauma can result in deviations in the axis of growth, premature fusion of the growth cartilage, and disturbances in osseous statics or dynamics. These traumas often go unnoticed, if the child does not mention them and there is no radiographic evidence.

Consider the example of a fall on the buttocks during childhood. The sacrum is not completely ossified until around age twenty. Application of traumatic kinetic energy to the growth cartilage can progressively disturb its growth or that of the related vertebra.

What are the consequences of this fall on vertebral statics and dynamics? What is the role of trauma in the genesis of certain types of spinal pain? We have seen numerous x-rays which demonstrate fusion of both vertebral stages. Rather than being congenital, this condition was apparently acquired following childhood trauma, as demonstrated by the fusion of the posterior arcs and confirmed by interview. The interview in such cases often reveals a violent fall on the back or buttocks which was not mentioned to parents and which the patient has never connected with her physical problems.

As osteopaths, we must pay special attention to children who have experienced significant trauma. We should ask patients about all traumatic events, even if they occurred well in the past. Tissue listening diagnosis and mobility tests are useful in this regard.

Articular restriction and trauma

Whereas major trauma may cause death of chondrocytes, lesser impact disturbs joint mechanics in more subtle ways.

We observe loss of joint mobility in patients every day, often resulting from trauma. Smaller joints are more vulnerable to this problem.

We believe that a "joint lesion" or restriction, as defined in osteopathy, can occur only as an effect of trauma. The muscular and ligamentous levels do not play a significant restrictive role. Mobility testing reveals a fixed and inelastic barrier in these cases.

Several scenarios are possible:

- localized drying of the two articular surfaces, modifying the axes of mobility
- interruption of the synovial liquid film
- indentation and loss of proper alignment of the surfaces
- loss of physical capacities (elasticity, plasticity) of the cartilaginous tissue
- jamming of bony segments, such as the sacrum between the ilia.

Alone or in combination, these elements disrupt articular mechanics through modification of curved surfaces, creation of areas of hypomobility, and changes in axes of mobility.

Capsular/synovial system

Fasciae

Connective tissues vary greatly in form and composition. Their "building blocks" are a basic ground substance and embryonic, reticular, interstitial, fibrous, and adipose connective tissues. The fibrous tissue with its high proportion of collagen fibers is most likely to retain memory of mechanical tension due to forces of collision. The viscoelasticity of the fascia allows storage of information induced by the energy of trauma.

Collagen, elastin, and reticulin fibers are biomechanically capable of reacting to and recording mechanical forces. The fluidity of the ground substance and the density of the various connective tissue fibers are affected by forces of collision. These two factors disturb the distensibility, elasticity, dampening, and restitution of energy of fasciae subjected to mechanical stress.

The tissues remember. The fasciae are slower to be "recorded" than muscle, a property which makes them more difficult to treat.

Ligaments and sprains

The resistant capsule is a constant formation in synovial articulations. It plays two crucial roles:

- containment and protection of the articular surfaces, synovial membrane, and synovial fluid
- mobility and stability; since the capsular tissue is only slightly elastic, it limits excessive movement.

A force which exceeds capsular resistance causes capsular distention or tearing, and sometimes an osseous break.

The ligaments play an essential role in the stability and mechanics of articulation. Their main function derives from their consistent length and limited extensibility. Typically, the ligaments reinforce the articular capsule in regions of greatest stress.

A sprain results when the force of trauma exceeds the mechanical resistance of a ligament.

- **Benign sprains** involve simple stretching or micro-ruptures of the ligament without a *dissolution of continuity*. Pain is intense because the nerve branches are intact, and can be triggered by slight mobilization of the joint or by palpation of the ligament. The micro-ruptures do not affect passive stability of the articulation.
- **Serious sprains** involve complete rupture of the ligament, by either avulsion of its bony insertion, or a tear in the middle of the fibrous region. Since the capsule is torn, there is always an ecchymosis, associated with hemarthrosis. Passive stability is lost, as seen by a pathological articular opening.

This articular instability which follows serious sprains has two components: objective laxity and a subjective sensation of "lack of reliability." It is important to distinguish these.

- **Objective laxity** can be constitutional or acquired following trauma. Acquired laxity reflects the absence of continuity and ineffectiveness of the ligament. It is not necessarily accompanied by a subjective sensation of instability.
- **Subjective instability** results from the absence of proprioceptive information, secondary to neuro-ligamentous rupture. The patient expresses this instability by fear or lack of confidence in the articulation.

This proprioceptive gap may be revealed by clinical examination following a serious sprain, independent of the degree of recuperation of stability.

Menisci and marginal folds

The marginal folds are inserted in the articular capsule and on the periphery of the concave articular surface. The menisci are attached mainly to the capsule, and are more mobile and fragile than the folds. Menisci may be detached, torn transversely or tangentially, or crushed during simple movements. The folds yield only to excessive stresses which accompany dislocations.

Symptomatology when these structures are detached or torn is of a free "foreign body" with characteristics dependent upon the specific articulation and the nature of the lesion. Cartilaginous deterioration can occur, associated with symptoms reflecting alteration of the fibro-cartilaginous structure.

Nervous system

When directly affected by trauma without being destroyed, the nervous system can either inhibit or facilitate the sensory and motor information it receives or sends.

Exteroceptive sensations derive from the skin and mucosa, while proprioceptive sensations come from the muscles, tendons, fasciae, and connective tissues. Autonomic innervation of viscera and their various envelopes, which are often damaged during trauma, is an additional factor.

Nerve impulses may be transmitted between neurons by chemical mediators different from the neurotransmitters which usually stimulate or inhibit. For certain sympathetic pathways, the neurons of the spinal cord are simultaneously cholinergic, noradrenergic, and serotonergic. There are still many gaps in our understanding of chemical mediation, which in our view make it impossible to clearly separate the sympathetic and parasympathetic systems. Trauma affects both catecholamines and serotonin, and these mediators may be able to modify neuronal chemical responses to various mechanical stimuli.

Neuromuscular spindles

These mechanoreceptors, located within the muscle, are stimulated by stretching. Their activity stops as soon as the muscle contracts. Some fibers of the neuromuscular spindles respond to momentary muscle stretching, while others register continuous stretching.

The spindles transmit their information to the motor neurons of the ventral horn of the spinal cord, which is a center of integration for motor regulation. Some of this information goes to the cerebellum via the spinocerebellar pathways.

Muscular, tendinous, fascial, or periosteal mechanical stimuli which are abnormal in either timing or intensity will "misinform" the ventral horn of the spinal cord and the cerebellar nuclei. As a result, muscular contractions, muscle tone, and general postural tone become poorly adapted, leading to less effective coordination of agonist and protagonist muscles. Regions with permanent muscle spasms are characterized by pain in addition to lack of muscular coordination.

Mechanoreceptors

Mechanoreceptors are sensitive to three types of stimulus: pressure, touch, and vibration. The free receptors (tactile corpuscles of Meissner, cells of Merckel, and corpuscles of Vater-Pacini, Krause, Golgi-Massoni, and Ruffini) are all affected by traumatic shock waves, even though they do not all function as typical mechanoreceptors.

Many of these mechanoreceptors are also thermodetectors (responding to infrared waves), and some may be sensitive to other electromagnetic wave lengths such as microwaves. There is still much we do not know about the capabilities of sensory organs.

Function of mechanoreceptors can be disrupted by mechanical trauma, in addition to changes in local electromagnetic field. Resulting sensory misinformation affects both local and general mechanical responses.

Coma

Coma is defined as a prolonged loss of consciousness. Its duration distinguishes it from a simple fainting spell. It is also different than sleep, from which the patient can be easily awakened and then recover complete consciousness within several seconds.

If coma is defined as an absence of consciousness, we must consider what we mean by this term. The various meanings of "consciousness" in everyday language reflect the interpretations of philosophers and neurobiologists: "I am aware of the situation," "I acted in accordance with my conscience," "He regained consciousness." These are three very different meanings.

Consciousness can be defined by its content (concepts) or by the ways in which this content can manifest itself (level of consciousness), in particular through language. Some comas involve total loss of conscious content. In others, which are more likely to be reversible, conscious content is intact but unable to be expressed.

Mechanisms of coma

The brain includes the brainstem and cerebral hemispheres. The cerebral cortex stores conscious content, and is activated by the mesencephalic *reticular formation*. This formation facilitates passage of sensory information in the thalamus toward the cerebral cortex, and also activates the cortex through diffuse nerve messages. The reticular formation thereby heightens the level of consciousness.

Functions which are not dependent upon consciousness are mediated by various subcortical structures, as in the following examples.

- The gray nuclei of the base and the brainstem control autonomic motor functions and muscle tone.
- Reflex movements are controlled by internal connections in the brainstem.
- The limbic system integrates the autonomic information coming from the viscera.
- The medulla oblongata controls respiration.

These autonomic functions and reflexes may be preserved during coma resulting from injury to the reticular formation or cortex. This type of coma is known as "persistent vegetative state." In contrast, when the brainstem is injured, these functions and reflexes are impaired and respiratory arrest occurs. Circulatory function may be maintained for some time if the patient is placed on a respirator, but this state is "beyond coma."

Etiology

Causes of coma can be assigned to several major categories:

- cerebral anoxia (lack of oxygen, typically seen in patients who are resuscitated after cardiac arrest)
- cerebral hemorrhage
- certain forms of poisoning
- hepatic or renal metabolic pathology leading to disruption of normal consciousness
- cranial trauma.

Whatever the cause, coma implies that the necessary nerve exchanges underlying storage or manifestation of consciousness are no longer being performed. Thus, there are two prerequisites for coma:

- loss of exchange of information between neurons

- the specific neurons involved are those responsible for storage or manifestation of conscious content.

TRAUMATIC COMA

Cranial trauma causes brain lesions, one of the major causes of coma. During sudden acceleration or deceleration of the head, as in whiplash, the impact of the brain against solid structures (cranial cavity, meninges) causes contusions in sensitive sites (immediate lesions). The mesencephalon can be damaged by its contact with the tentorium cerebelli. Specific regions of the cerebral hemispheres are subject to contusion depending on the direction of movement. Lesion of the reticular formation accounts for loss of consciousness following trauma, as described above.

Edema from traumatic head injury can lead to displacement of the brain and engagement of cerebral tissue in the orifice of the tentorium cerebelli. Obstruction of the aqueduct of Silvius then interferes with CSF flow, causing increase of subtentorial intracranial pressure.

Oxygenation of neurons in the brain depends on cerebral perfusion pressure (difference between arterial and intracranial pressure). *If this pressure differential disappears, the neurons are no longer oxygenated.* Moreover, movement toward the base of the brainstem as above interferes with normal vascular structure and causes hemorrhage and swelling of the brainstem, with risk of anoxia in the regions beneath the tentorium cerebelli. In the absence of treatment to reduce intracranial pressure, major cerebral edema can therefore cause destruction of both cortex and brainstem tissue, leading to brain death.

Visceral system

Study of the pathophysiology of visceral lesions helps us to better understand results obtained by visceral manipulation. Visceral trauma, unless severe, is often neglected in conventional medical practice. This is unfortunate, as it is the key to understanding many patients' problems. There are both direct and indirect effects on the organs.

Direct effects of trauma

STRETCHING OF THE SYSTEM OF ATTACHMENTS

The ligaments and fasciae attached to visceral organs contain sensitive proprioceptors, which provide local and central sensory information on organ movement, volume, and weight. They are:

- mechanoreceptors
- volume receptors
- pressure receptors.

Sudden stretching of these receptors during trauma can either inhibit or overstimulate them. They consequently send misinformation to local, regional, and central nerve centers ("proprioceptive deprogramming"). Normal feedback motor functions are correspondingly disrupted, and the organ is impaired in its blood and lymph circulation, becomes congested, and loses some of its function and vitality.

INTRINSIC INTERNAL LESIONS

The forces of traumatic collision can cause actual fissures or fractures to solid visceral organs (e.g., kidneys, liver, spleen, pancreas), as verified in dissections.

In the kidney, for example, post-traumatic hematuria causes a parenchymatous lesion. This is usually micro-hematuria, which gives the urine a dark color. Ask the patient if urine was dark in the days following the trauma. In other organs (e.g., lung) we may note internal disseminated lesions at points where forces of collision are concentrated.

EXTRINSIC INTERNAL LESIONS

During traumatic impact, the visceral organs may strike into or be struck by bony elements. For example, the bladder may crash into the pelvic girdle, or the liver into the ribcage, with resulting contusions or dissections which cause significant bleeding and edema. In such cases, the patient often exhibits elevated temperature and hypotension.

ORGAN DISPLACEMENT

Surprisingly, little attention is paid to organ displacement in conventional medicine, except in extreme cases of violent trauma. We once saw an accident victim in the hospital whose liver had torn the diaphragm and pleura, and moved into the right hemithorax. More commonly, certain organs (particularly the kidney) are displaced from normal anatomic position.

Abdominal organs can be displaced upward or downward by a fall on the buttocks, hyperpressure of traumatic origin, or concentration of the forces of collision. When an organ is displaced several millimeters or even centimeters below its normal position in the abdomen, it loses part of the beneficial action of diaphragmatic attraction. Venous, lymphatic, and arterial circulation are affected. Without treatment, the organ becomes more congested and heavier, less functional, less supported, and therefore migrates even lower down.

We have seen intravenous urographies in which the right kidney is clearly visualized in the lesser pelvis, without this fact being mentioned in the patient's summary. How can an organ displaced more than a dozen centimeters from its normal position continue to function effectively?

The bladder is capable of moving 1-2cm laterally, which is sufficient to cause incontinence. We have also noted small displacements of the liver. Dolichogastry (elongation) or abnormal tension of the peri-hiatal fibers may occur in the stomach.

During visceral manipulation, the hands are pressed into the abdomen and under the thorax in a search for tissue lesions and visceral restrictions. This may reveal lesions that were not evident on gross palpation or x-ray. It is difficult to compare the various forms of imaging technology with manual exploration, as each can reveal problems not revealed by the other.

Indirect effects of trauma

LESIONS CAUSED BY STRESS

Whereas trauma creates direct visceral lesions, indirect lesions are induced by stress. The visceral system is the preferred target of somatization. Trauma may affect the stomach both in its system of attachments (direct lesion) and by development of an ulcer from psychological stress reaction (indirect lesion). Although objective proof is difficult, many gastroenterologists agree with us regarding the high frequency of post-traumatic ulcers.

We once had a patient who complained, following an automobile accident, of severe left intercostal pain which worsened in the evening. We know that nocturnal pain is a sign of visceral problems. Listening tests and manual thermal diagnosis kept returning us to the level of the lesser gastric curvature, between the pylorus and Oddi's sphincter. Various imaging and biochemical tests proved negative.

The left intercostal pain increased and the patient's left shoulder also became painful. His general state suddenly declined, with appearance of pallor, nausea, loss of appetite, excessive fatigue, and weight loss. He turned out to have a "hidden" stomach ulcer which had perforated the stomach and attacked the pancreas, causing acute pancreatitis. The initial symptom which brought him to our office had been simple intercostal pain!

Vertebral lesions

It is not necessary for us to cover the topic of vertebral lesions here, as they play a central role in osteopathy and are widely discussed. Damage to a vertebra, of course, impairs afferent and efferent nervous connections to the corresponding organ. The organ, therefore, is less well supplied with blood and slowly loses its vitality and immune protection. Its loss of normal function progressively affects related organs and the entire body.

Vascular systems

Arterio-venous system

Vascular problems following a collision may affect primarily the superior cervicothoracic vessels. These problems are usually due to arterial spasms resulting from nervous system stimulation. Coronary spasms may cause transient coronary insufficiency.

Numerous arteries are affected by cranial trauma, in particular the vertebral artery (see below) and meningeal arteries, which are greatly impacted by injury of the dura mater. The subclavian arteries are less affected by vasoconstriction than by decrease in rate, which is due largely to abnormal tension in the surrounding soft tissue (subclavius and scalene muscles, pleurocervical, conoid, and trapezoid ligaments).

Vertebral artery

The importance of the vertebral artery is demonstrated by the many problems in its perfusion areas caused by reduction of its flow, and the improvement seen after treatment of surrounding muscles and fasciae.

Anatomical considerations

Both the left and right vertebral arteries have an outside diameter of 3-4mm, but the left one often has a larger lumen. The left vertebral artery goes higher, more internally, and more posteriorly than the right one.

The *transverse groove* is delimited:

- in back and in front by the intertransverse muscles
- internally by the intervertebral disk
- externally by the attachments of the scalene muscles to the transverse processes.

The vertebral artery in the transverse groove is related laterally to its vein, and posteriorly to the sino-vertebral nerve and intertransverse muscles. Superiorly, the vertebral artery is hidden by the lateral occipito-atloid ligament and muscles inserting on the transverse process of the atlas *(Fig. 3-1)*.

The first posterior intertransverse separates the vertebral artery from the large oblique muscle extending from the spinous process of the axis to the transverse process of the atlas.

The vertebral artery passes through the epidural space linked to the roots of the first cervical nerve. The dura mater attached to the artery is drawn by it into the spinal canal.

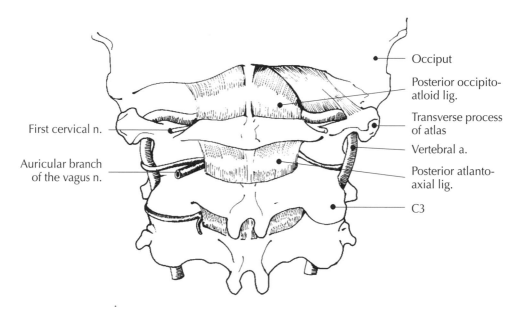

First cervical n.

Auricular branch of the vagus n.

Occiput

Posterior occipito-atloid lig.

Transverse process of atlas

Vertebral a.

Posterior atlanto-axial lig.

C3

Fig. 3-1: Elbow of the vertebral artery

COMPRESSION OF THE VERTEBRAL ARTERY

The artery may be pushed back or compressed in cases of uncarthrosis, posterior interapophysial arthrosis, or disk arthrosis.

Herniated disks are usually associated with sensory difficulties. In some cases, compression of the vertebral artery causes other symptoms.

Intertransverse mechanical problems irritate the sympathetic nervous system, which sends the vertebral artery into spasm (reflex vasoconstriction). Spasm of the intertransverse muscles is also possible, which modifies the relations of the transverse canal with the vertebral artery.

When the dura mater is stretched by trauma, it may affect the pathway of the vertebral artery in the first intraspinal segment. There are fibers connecting the adventitia of the artery to the surrounding dura.

VERTEBRAL ARTERY COLLATERALS

Decreased flow through the vertebral artery in turn reduces flow through its collaterals, ultimately affecting blood supply to the medulla.

The cervical collaterals are subdivided into four branches:

- muscular
- spinal (for the vertebrae, spinal cord, and its envelopes)
- articular
- meningeal.

The intracranial collaterals are:

- posterior meningeal artery (the continuation of the vertebral after it has traversed the dura mater)
- anterior and posterior spinal arteries
- posterior and inferior cerebellar arteries.

PROTECTION OF THE VERTEBRAL ARTERY

Studies by Claude Manelfe (1989) support our viewpoint that the vertebral arteries play a primary role in vascularizing the primary autonomic centers of the brainstem. The arteries are protected by:

- the transverse foramen, where the artery is covered by a venous plexus providing passive hydraulic protection
- the uncinate process, a lateral elevation of the upper surface of the cervical vertebra, particularly well-developed posteriorly.

The uncinate process creates a push toward the top of the lateral part of the disk, by avoiding lateral bulging in certain movements *(Fig. 3-2)*. Such bulging can compress the vertebral artery and reduce its flow.

At its entry to the skull, the vertebral artery is affected by movements of rotation, sidebending, and extension. With movements (primarily extension) in which the artery is stretched and compressed, there is some risk of localized decreased perfusion. In general, flow is kept constant in all head positions because of the union of the vertebral arteries in a single basilar artery. The risk of cerebellar hypocirculation is greatest when the arms are in the air and the head extended. Based on our experience, if cerebellar circulation is disturbed, even if it is quickly reestablished, it can take about one month for the cerebellum to fully recover its function.

Dissections of arteries of the neck

It is important to know the symptoms of arterial dissections in the neck, even though not all cases are of traumatic origin. Congenital weaknesses of the wall of neck arteries can place a patient's life in danger during an accident, or poorly executed manipulation.

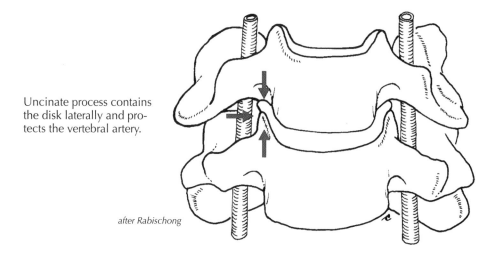

Uncinate process contains
the disk laterally and protects the vertebral artery.

after Rabischong

Fig. 3-2: Passage of the vertebral artery in the transverse cervical canal

Dissections are most commonly seen in the extracranial pathways of the internal carotid and vertebral arteries, less commonly in the intracranial pathways of these same arteries.

ANATOMY AND PATHOLOGY

Dissections or aneurysms are due to cleavage of the arterial wall by a hematoma, causing concentric clefts in the vascular linings. A hematoma causes both an increase in the outside diameter of the artery and a reduction of its lumen.

Mechanism

Two mechanisms have been proposed for arterial dissections:

- intimal tear, allowing blood to accumulate inside the intima
- intramural hematoma, causing a gap in the intima.

In contrast to an aortic dissection in which there is a cleavage of the arterial wall creating a true or false groove, dissections of the arteries of the neck cause a hematoma which increases the outside diameter of the artery, with attendant reduction in lumen width.

Progression of the dissection occurs in the direction of arterial flow. Stenosis of the arterial lumen causes occlusion. An aneurysm may occur when the dissection extends to the adventitia.

Location

Dissections of the vertebral artery are most commonly located at the superior exit of the transverse groove, with the atlantoaxial segment most involved. More rarely, they are located at the entry to the transverse canal in C6, and even more rarely, intracranially. In 60% of cases, dissections of the vertebral arteries are bilateral. In the case of fibromuscular dysplasia, tearing of the vertebral artery can accompany that of the renal arteries.

Tearing of the basilar artery is very rare and serious. In more than 30% of cases this causes meningeal hemorrhage.

Because of the possible presence of dissections at the exit of the transverse canal, we must be very careful when performing high cervical manipulations. It is prudent to avoid aggressive cervical manipulations with a hyperextended occiput when the technique includes major rotation of the occiput/C1 on C2-C3. A small osseous obstacle or adhesion on the intra-transverse vertebral artery can create an abnormal arterial mechanical stress with a risk of tearing. Dissections of the vertebral artery may be extended to the carotid.

PATHOGENESIS

Mechanical and traumatic causes

Many activities or mechanical factors promote the development of vertebral artery dissections: stressful physical activities (bicycle, jogging, sailing, obstetrical labor, violent or repeated coughing), constricting positions of the occipitocervical region (yoga, hairstyling, painting the ceiling), and positions stressing the extended neck.

The risk is increased when, in addition to cervical extension, the arms are extended. Many people fixing up their homes fall from a ladder without knowing why after assuming this position. What has happened is a momentary slowdown or stoppage of vertebral artery flow to the cerebellum, resulting in loss of balance. This position (arms outstretched, head back) almost always causes compression of the subclavian arteries in the cervicothoracic junction, which induces a slowdown of vertebral artery blood flow.

The subclavian artery in the thoracic outlet is usually compressed, without circulatory ramifications, when the arm is abducted and externally rotated. However, some types of repeated exertion with the arms extended, such as sailing, can create a micropneumothorax, which is difficult to demonstrate. This causes a slowdown of subclavian artery blood flow, which is also disturbed in the thoracic outlet by abnormal mechanical tension of the cervicopleural ligaments and neck muscles.

Arthrosis of the cervical spine

In the event of uncarthrosis or cervical disk arthrosis, the vertebral artery can easily become misaligned in the transverse canal. Movement of the cervical spine, repeated coughing, or a powerful sneeze can create pathogenic mechanical stress of the vertebral artery, which is capable of creating longitudinal tearing.

Arterial structural abnormalities

These include arterial sinuosity and flexing, narrowing of the arterial lumen, and kinking syndrome (thoracic aorta plaited by a short arterial ligament).

PATIENTS AT RISK

Predisposing factors include:

- arterial hypertension, particularly a hypertensive crisis
- intense migraines
- smoking and taking birth control pills
- congenital arterial weakness
- sequelae of infection

- fibromuscular dysplasia
- disease of the arterial wall
- Marfan's syndrome
- cervical trauma.

Patients most at risk are adults around 40 years of age. In 10% of cases, there are causal or predisposing factors such as those listed above. We believe that craniocervical trauma is a greater factor in vertebral artery dissection than is commonly recognized. Many patients don't remember trauma experienced in childhood or adolescence.

In conclusion, the classic at-risk patient is around 40 years of age and a smoker. If female, she takes birth control pills. The patient has experienced one or several cranio-cervical traumas, engages in physical activities which extend and stress the cervical spine, and exhibits degenerative changes in the cervical spine. She may complain of dizziness, instability, nausea, or headaches.

SYMPTOMATOLOGY

Prodromal signs of vertebral artery dissections can appear hours or days before the actual onset.

The most common symptom is neck pain with temporal radiation that resembles a migraine or facial vascular pain. (*Note:* Headaches of cervical origin begin in the posterior area and spread to the frontal regions. Only very rarely do they radiate toward the face or have a pulsatile quality. There may also be dizziness, a temporary reeling gait, and a pulsatile tinnitus.)

Horner's syndrome

Horner's syndrome (or Bernard-Horner's syndrome) refers to a combination of unilateral ptosis (drooping of the upper eyelid), contraction of the pupil, anhidrosis (deficiency of facial sweating), and enophthalmos (backward displacement of the eyeball). It is due to a lesion of either the cervical sympathetic chain or its central pathways. This can be a sign of dissection of the internal carotid, especially if accompanied by intense headache.

NATURAL HISTORY

The natural progression of this problem has a favorable outcome in 70% of cases, but in some serious cases the end result is quadraplegia or even death. In the presence of Horner's syndrome, a spontaneous regression occurs in only 30% of cases (Lavieille et. al, 1986). In its acute phase, angiography reveals a functional occlusion of the artery which can spontaneously regain patency.

Changes in CSF pressure

We have had 20 patients with documented changes in CSF pressure. Since the symptoms and complaints were highly variable, most of these patients were placed by specialists in the large "catch-basin" of patients deemed to have a primarily psychological disorder! It is generally difficult to relate specific symptoms to a decrease or increase in CSF pressure.

The brain functions best when CSF pressure is 12-15cm H_2O. Recall that CSF pressure is responsible for the fact that a brain which weighs 1.2kg in air has an effective weight of 40g! It is obviously important that cranial CSF pressure remain constant. If CSF pressure drops, the effective weight of the brain increases. Compression of the brain tends to stimulate it, increasing the secretion rate of endorphins, serotonin, and, to a lesser extent, adrenalin.

SYMPTOMS OF CSF PRESSURE CHANGES

Excessive CSF pressure is characterized by torpor, plus various combinations of somnolence, nausea, dizziness, sensory paresthesias, and problems with vision, hearing, balance, memory, cognitive acuity, or behavior. The symptoms vary according to the degree of trauma. Patients presenting with fatigue and loss of memory after a simple case of whiplash may have high CSF pressure.

Low CSF pressure is usually due to leakage of CSF after the dura mater has been cleaved longitudinally by trauma or spinal tap. However, it is very difficult to show direct evidence of such longitudinal dissections. Rather, leakage of fluid is indicated by the symptoms and decrease of CSF pressure. Symptoms of low CSF pressure include dizziness, lack of balance, sudden anxiety, and paresis, mainly of the lower limbs.

Note: We believe that in some cases of cranial or spinal trauma, there are micro-leakages of CSF which are not revealed by conventional medical examination. Following vertebral trauma, such leakages are due to longitudinal dura mater tearing caused by intracavity osseous irregularities. In most of these cases, healing is rapid and spontaneous. Sometimes, however, the patient suffers for months or even years from subjective problems which may be attributed to post-traumatic depression. Manual listening can uncover this type of problem.

POST-SPINAL TAP SYNDROME

This syndrome often produces symptoms similar to those of a patient who has undergone cranial trauma. In certain cases, especially when the patient has undergone many spinal punctures, a break may occur in the dura mater with leakage of CSF and decrease of cerebral blood flow.

Lowering of CSF pressure leads to ptosis ("heaviness") of the brain, along with strong dura mater tension. The patient may exhibit headache, diffuse pain, nausea, vomiting, and stiffness of the neck or entire spine, sometimes resembling acute cervical or lower back pain. This group of symptoms resembles that of meningeal syndrome (nausea, vomiting, stiffness). Diffuse paresthesias, vagotonia with pallor, and profuse perspiration often complete the clinical picture.

Note: Headaches of post-spinal tap syndrome characteristically increase in standing position and decrease in supine position.

According to many neurologists, treatment for post-spinal tap syndrome calls for drinking three or more liters of liquid per day to promote CSF production. The patient should lie in supine position, which both decreases dura mater traction and indirectly increases cranial pressure. Despite compartmentalization, all bodily intracavity pressures are interdependent.

A similar mechanism operates in patients with a type of dizziness triggered by a change from seated or standing to supine position. This dizziness does not occur if the patient goes from standing to prone position. Abdominal compression must play a role, but the phenomenon takes place even without abdominal support.

We have been summoned to hospitals and clinics many times by anesthesiologists who were unable to help their patients recover from the side effects of a spinal tap, that is, cervical or lower back pain, or persistent headache, often after epidurals given during labor.

In these cases there was always significant restriction of T8-T9 (where the spinal canal is narrowest and the spinal cord is most compressed). Manipulation of these two vertebra leads to immediate and lasting relief of symptoms. Many patients had been taking analgesics and anti-inflammatory drugs for several days. Our manipulations relaxed dura mater traction and perhaps improved circulation of radicular and spinal arteries.

Note: We advise against lumbar puncture for patients with scoliosis, spinal cord problems, migraine headaches, or past cranial or vertebral trauma.

Post-traumatic sensory deficits

In Chapter 2 we emphasized the role of the cranial openings in distribution and dampening of internal pressure. In the case of trauma, the inner ear is under significant pressure, which has a major impact on hearing and balance.

Effects of trauma on hearing

During acceleration and deceleration from cranial impact, the skull and its contents undergo deformations which affect the walls of the inner ear. The endolymphatic fluid is abruptly displaced, causing a cochlear concussion. The sensory cells of the cochlea are no longer normally stimulated by the fluid waves caused by sound vibrations, and auditory perception is altered.

Vertebral artery and hearing

We have often noted hearing injury associated with worsening of memory in our patients who have experienced whiplash. We believe that this is due to reduced blood flow through the vertebral artery and its branch, the cochlear artery. The sensory cells of the cochlea , which depend on constant blood supply, cease to respond normally.

Doctors Pierre Lucas and Michel Stehman of the Free University of Brussels believe that hypoxia or anoxia of the sensory cochlear cells are always accompanied by middle ear problems.

Tinnitus

This is a frequent sequela of craniocervical trauma. It can be due to constriction of the arteries of the middle and inner ear, which creates a sort of pulsatile whirring, or random and continuous stimulation of the labyrinthine cells. These stimuli cause continuous cavernous background noise, as if the patient were in a cave. The sympathetic nervous system seems to be the cause. Suppression of tinnitus is often difficult.

Balance

The membranous labyrinth is affected by the forces of collision. The endolymph no longer properly stimulates the sensory cells situated at the level of the crista ampularis, semi-circular canals, and membranes of the saccule and utricule. Consequently, the vestibular nuclei do not receive proper sensory input for decoding and distribution to the body, particularly in regard to cerebellar control. The cerebellum normally consolidates labyrinthine, visual, kinesthetic, and thermal information which is used to provide motor output for correct balance. In post-traumatic syndromes, some of the sensory inputs no longer yield proper responses.

VESTIBULE

The vestibule (central, oval portion of the bony labyrinth) is one of the oldest of the sensory organs in mammalian evolution. It has several special characteristics.

- Its activation is unconscious and automatic.
- It is always active, even during sleep.
- It is connected to the muscular reflex system.
- Its reaction time is extremely brief.
- Its stimulation threshold is very low.

For example, unusual types of acceleration lead to motion sickness due primarily to stimulation of the labyrinth. Motion sickness is characterized by nausea, vomiting, pallor, sweating, faintness, and vasovagal syndrome (peripheral vasodilation, brady-cardia, and hypotension due to stimulation of the vagus nerve).

Motion sickness may persist in mild form for months or years after unusual trauma. The forces of acceleration and deceleration can "deprogram" the sensory cells of the membranous labyrinth. The clinical signs above, which are prominent at first, diminish over time. The patient feels a malaise that he no longer attributes to the accident. These lingering symptoms, acting at a subconscious level, may produce chronic anxiety or depression.

Sense of smell

Certain people lose the sense of smell completely or partially (anosmia) following trauma. Anosmia also affects perception of taste. Food seems tasteless, even though the four types of taste buds in the mouth (sweet, salty, bitter, sour) are still functional. Numerous factors besides trauma can cause anosmia, including coryza (acute hay fever), neoplasms, and viral or bacterial infections. Causes of anosmia must be clearly defined before treatment is begun.

In cranial trauma, anosmia is not always due to fracture of the cribriform plate of the ethmoid bone. Occipital or parietal trauma caused by rebound after impact can damage the tracts of the olfactory bulb.

Chapter Four:
Clinical Complaints
Related to Trauma

Table of Contents

Clinical Complaints
Related to Trauma

Migraines and Other Headaches

Headache is one of the most common symptoms for which patients consult us. Here we differentiate migraines from other types of headaches, although in our daily practice this distinction is sometimes blurred.

Migraines

The suffering and costs from migraine headaches have tremendous social impact. In France, three to four million people suffer from migraines; two-thirds are women. The mechanisms and causes of migraine are complex and varied.

Mechanisms of migraines

CIRCULATORY SYSTEM

During a migraine attack, overall cerebral circulation may decrease, and subsequently increase. Stimulation of certain brainstem nuclei by the trigeminal nerve (see below) may trigger these vasomotor phenomena.

Vasodilation

Electrical stimulation of vessels supplying the scalp (superficial temporal artery) and extracerebral dura mater (middle meningeal artery) is painful, whereas stimulation of the surrounding soft tissues is not. The pain is thought to be due in part to arterial vasodilation, which is often preceded by vasoconstriction. Inflammation of arterial walls, with vasodilation and edema from vasoactive peptides and other pain-inducing substances, also contribute to intensity of the pain.

NERVOUS SYSTEM

The *trigeminal nerve* carries pain messages from the inflamed arterial wall to the brainstem, triggering migraine pain. Headaches may be related to mechanical irritation of the sensitive nerve endings of the meninges. In rats, meningeal nerve endings are chemosensitive, and chemical stimulation may sensitize them to mechanical stimuli. In humans, the intracranial hypersensitivity characteristic of certain types of headaches, and the shooting pain of migraines, may be explained in this way.

Chemistry of body fluids

Biochemical changes of blood and tissue fluids associated with headaches are varied, and poorly understood. Increased levels of the following have been recorded during migraines:

- serotonin
- platelets
- catecholamines (noradrenaline, dopamine, tyramine)
- histamine
- free fatty acids
- prostaglandins.

Causes of migraines

Chronic migraine sufferers tend to be hyperactive. Often a slight stimulus can trigger an attack. We can view these people as having low "migrainogenic" thresholds, and high vascular reactivity to catecholamines.

FOOD CAUSES

Some foods are clearly more migrainogenic than others. Predisposition to migraines may be related to particular food combinations, plus time of the week (some people only get migraines during the weekend) or stage of menstrual cycle. For example, eating creamed salmon, then chocolate, and washing it down with white wine during the pre-menstrual stage is almost guaranteed to cause migraine in a predisposed woman. Some soft cheeses containing tyramine or phenylethylamine can trigger migraines.

Colored *alcohols* are more likely to be migrainogenic than clear alcohols such as gin and vodka. White wine causes migraines, but this seems to be due to the high sulfite content rather than the alcohol itself.

Milk *chocolate* is more migrainogenic than dark chocolate, perhaps due to the presence of cooked cream.

Besides white wine, many common foods contain sulfites as preservatives. These include beer, cider, apple juice, carrots, mashed potatoes, and dried apricots. Tell your migraine patients to avoid any food or drug containing sulfites.

HORMONAL CAUSES

Migraines are more likely during the premenstrual stage of the cycle, especially when triggered by certain foods or other factors.

We have had little success in treating migraine-prone women whose attacks stop during pregnancy. Estrogen level has been correlated with triggering of migraines. The headache coincides with the drop in estrogen just before onset of menstruation. Menopause "cures" half of all female migraine sufferers.

PSYCHOLOGICAL FACTORS

Patients suffering from depression often have migraines. We believe that these are due to the associated hypersensitivity and hyperreactivity, rather than the depression itself. In addition, most antidepressant medications cause problems with liver metabolism, thereby increasing the likelihood of migraines. Not all depression patients suffer from migraines; other migrainogenic factors as above greatly increase the likelihood.

Types of migraines

CLASSIC MIGRAINE WITH AURA

A migraine "aura" reflects some sort of cerebral dysfunction. It begins within 5-20 minutes of the migraine and fades away in less than an hour. There are various types of aura:

- visual: a lacy or luminous image superimposed on the visual field, leaving a scotoma (blind spot) as it disappears
- sensory: paresthesia (abnormal sensation of burning, prickling, bugs crawling on the skin, etc.), itching on half of the face or body, feeling of numbness
- verbal: troubles with elocution, missing words, jargon aphasia.

MIGRAINE WITHOUT AURA

Attacks are preceded by prodrome including such symptoms as fatigue, sleeplessness, slight behavioral problems, and decreased appetite. The migraine appears quickly, and affects the suborbital, frontal, and less often the occipital areas. The patient may awaken early in the morning with the attack. It is one-sided, pulsatile, and often causes photophobia, nausea, vomiting, or a state of prostration. The migraine may last from a few hours up to three days.

ATYPICAL AURAS

Besides the typical migraine auras described above, there are a few rarer types:

- prolonged aura, lasting more than one hour and less than one week. May be caused by local ischemia or intracerebral hematoma.
- hemiparesic migraine: hemiparesis (weakness on one side of the body) is present and often found in a close relative as well
- basilar migraine: related to dysfunction of the brainstem or occipital lobes. Associated with visual problems, dysarthria (impaired speech articulation), tinnitus, partial hearing loss, double vision, impaired memory or consciousness, bilateral paresis (incomplete paralysis), paresthesia, or dizziness.

Trauma and migraines

In our practice we see many migraine cases which seem to involve trauma. Collisions or impacts of various types can be aggravating factors in an environment which is already migrainogenic.

Headaches caused by trauma typically have an occipital or nuchal (back of the neck) manifestation, and a low cervical origin (C5-C6-C7).

We sometimes see one-sided headaches that are not really migraines, but rather due to high vertebral (C1-C2-C3) or cranial restrictions. These disappear after one or two sessions, whereas true migraines improve gradually rather than disappear completely.

Other headaches

Other types of headache differ from migraines in location, intensity, and complexity.

Location and origin

Non-migraine headaches often begin with nuchal and occipital pain, which migrates slowly toward the anterior cerebral regions, unilaterally or bilaterally, and ends up in the sinuses, frontal, periorbital, or more rarely, zygomatic region.

The origin of non-migraine headaches is frequently mechanical (skull, cervical, upper thoracic, sacral segments) or vascular (particularly arterial hypertension).

Note: Headaches of mechanical origin usually start out posterior, then radiate toward the median and anterior cranial regions. They are rarely facial. *They are not accompanied by a rise in temperature, vomiting, strabismus, or a sensation of impending danger.* These symptoms often indicate either a serious intracranial infection or a tumor.

Time of occurrence

Typical times of occurrence are:

- cyclic, at fixed times (neuralgic origin)
- nocturnal (vascular hypertension)
- erratic, sudden, and intense (neuralgic origin)
- early morning (digestive origin, related to alcohol and/or tobacco toxicity).

There are obviously exceptions to this general classification. A patient with neck pain who sleeps on a bad pillow may have early morning headache unrelated to the digestive system or alcohol/tobacco usage.

Causes

POST-TRAUMATIC HEADACHES

These may appear following any type of trauma to the head. If a headache immediately following an accident is accompanied by malaise, syncope, paresthesia, or brief paresis, check for loss of CSF and hypotension. These symptoms are common after a lumbar puncture (see Chapter 3).

ARTERIAL HYPERTENSION

Hypertension causes diffuse, predominantly occipital headaches in early evening or early morning. Confusingly, hypotension can cause the same symptoms.

ENDOCRANIAL COMPRESSION

Endocranial compression causes serious headaches accompanied by symptoms such as projectile vomiting, bradycardia, papilledema (edema of the optic disk), and paralysis of the sixth cranial nerve.

OTHER CAUSES

Other causes of non-migraine headache include drugs (more commonly than many physicians realize), endocrine disorders, and joint problems.

Neck Pain

This is a common and well-studied complaint. Not all cases are of traumatic or mechanical origin. We will briefly review some important types of neck pain to aid in differential diagnosis.

Post-traumatic neck pain

Neck pain and other effects of cervical trauma have fairly specific symptomatology.

Local signs

DELAYED APPEARANCE OF SYMPTOMS

Following trauma, neck pain usually does not appear immediately. For a day or so the victim is in a state of dulled sensitivity. Only after this state has dissipated does the pain manifest itself.

LOWER CERVICAL PAIN

Pain is typically focused around C4 through C7, at the level of the supraspinal and interspinal ligaments, intertransverse muscles, and laminae.

OCCIPITAL PAIN

The occipital attachments of neck muscles are also irritated. In particular, palpation reveals several tender points on the occipital attachment of the trapezius.

PAIN IS RELIEVED BY REST

Post-traumatic neck pain is reduced if the patient finds a position which relaxes the muscles and ligaments of the cervical/thoracic area. In contrast, neck pain of infectious or rheumatic origin is sometimes aggravated by rest.

LIMITATION OF MOVEMENT

Rotation is usually limited more on one side than the other. Advise the patient to move her neck in the nonpainful direction, and lie on the back, with a thin cushion under the occiput.

DIFFICULTY OF EXTENSION

In some cases of post-traumatic neck pain, extension is dangerous as well as difficult. At a certain degree of hyperextension, the patient finds it impossible to hold up the head, and pain becomes severe. Extension causes a reduction in diameter of the vertebral artery lumen, and the pain may cause reflex spasm of the arterial walls, with immediate sensation of nausea and dizziness.

General signs

Less localized symptoms associated with post-traumatic neck pain include the following.

HEADACHES THAT BEGIN POSTERIORLY

Patients may describe vague headache pain of nuchal origin, which later becomes occipital and finally frontal. These headaches are rarely migraines. They may be strongest in the occipital and lateral parietal regions, and bilateral at the frontal level.

AN IMPRESSION OF FUZZINESS AND FLOATING

The patient may have sensations of floating, or as if the head is "full of cotton." These sensations are probably of cerebellar origin. The patient feels as if all information has been filtered and attenuated, and as if she is not in direct contact with reality.

POSITIONAL DIZZINESS

The patient is subject to dizziness, which she experiences only upon changing from prone to upright position or vice versa, or when turning the head too rapidly. This dizziness may be confused with the "cotton" feeling described above.

FEELING OF INSTABILITY

There is no real functional problem with balance, but the patient feels unstable, as if slightly inebriated. For example, she feels uneasy walking down a narrow corridor.

SENSATION OF FATIGUE

This is not extreme fatigue like that seen in restrictions of the kidney or spleen, but the patient cannot completely relax, and sleep is disturbed by neck pain and post-traumatic stress.

ABSENCE OF FEVER AND NODE ENLARGEMENT

Cervical trauma *per se* does not cause fever or enlargement of nodes. However, we have seen many patients who developed a slight fever and inflamed cervical and subclavicular nodes following an accident. Further interview revealed the presence of ear/nose/throat infection, or more generalized infection such as mononucleosis, prior to the accident. Such differential diagnosis is difficult since patients tend to attribute their symptoms to the accident.

Of the thousands of patients we have seen following head/neck trauma, less than a dozen showed a slight increase in temperature, which could have been due to contusions and resulting edema. Conceivably, cranial trauma might disturb the thermoregulatory control centers of the hypothalamus.

Torticollis

In children

We see many young children who consult for torticollis (unnatural position of the head due to contracted cervical muscles) in the absence of recent CNS shock or trauma. *These cases are almost always caused by infections, which may be undetected!* Manipulation is contraindicated, and carries the risk of creating a vertebral sprain. Inform the child's parents that around ten years of age, a child's immune defenses are relatively weak. This is the age when many unnecessary appendectomies are performed.

Acute torticollis in children may be accompanied by inflammation of the cervical lymph nodes and surrounding connective tissues. In these cases, look carefully for enlargement of lateral cervical, subclavicular, and axillary nodes. Think first of an acute sore throat or dental problem.

In adults

Torticollis in adults has many possible causes besides trauma: dental pathology, arthrosis, arthritis, cold, or an infection.

DENTAL PATHOLOGY

Upon visiting a ski resort in the Alps, some patients develop neck pain and cervicobrachial neuralgia, which disappear upon return to lower altitudes. These signs are due to variations in barometric pressure, which influence the spaces inside teeth, and edema surrounding nerve roots during inflammation.

ARTHROSIS

This osteoarticular attack begins with degeneration of the cartilage, then changes in subchondral bone associated with secondary synovitis. Cartilage is composed of a matrix of hydrophilic proteoglycans interspersed with collagenous fibers and chondrocytes. Cartilage contains 75% water, accounting for its viscoelastic properties and susceptibility to degeneration.

Regeneration of cartilage requires pressure. Plaster cast immobilization of a joint causes the cartilage to deteriorate because of a lack of alternation between pressure and rest, in addition to muscular wasting.

Post-traumatic arthrosis

In cases of abnormal mechanical tension transmitted by muscles and tendons, there is a type of intracartilaginous increased pressure which causes long-term degeneration of the cartilage. This is in contrast to structural arthrosis, such as the congenital weakness of the cartilage in chondrocalcinosis (presence of calcium pyrophosphate), epiphyseal osteonecrosis, or synovitis.

This phenomenon is common following whiplash when the cervical sprain gradually causes abnormal mechanical tension of the lower cervical vertebrae. Ligamentous tension and cartilaginous pressure around C5 and C6 is modified. Abnormal ligamentous tension can create a syndesmophyte (bony outgrowth from a ligament). Traumatic injury of a ligament or muscle can be confirmed by ligamentous calcifications visible on x-ray. Usually, anterolateral elements are most affected.

Pathophysiology

Excessive pressure transmitted by articular tissues and periarticular soft tissues causes expansion of proteoglycans and overhydration of cartilage. Swollen cartilage is the first biochemical manifestation of post-traumatic arthrosis. Biomechanical characteristics of the cartilage are altered. Cushioning of pressure on top of subchondral bone is less effective, the cartilage is condensed, and reactive osteophytosis may develop. Fissured areas, fibrillations, and ulcerations are seen under the microscope.

Phases of post-traumatic arthrosis

In the *reactive phase*, mechanical pressure causes proliferation and increased activity of chondrocytes, increasing synthesis of hydrophilic proteoglycans and collagen fibers.

In the *destructive phase*, chondrocytes become less active, then degenerate. The matrix loses viscoelasticity and the ability to resist mechanical tension. This process is followed by arthrosis.

Arthritis

Acute arthritis

This is characterized by acute neck pain without precipitating trauma. Some abnormalities are seen on biomedical exams. X-rays of the neck often reveal calcifications on the transverse ligament behind the odontoid process.

Arthritis of malignant origin

Certain malignant conditions can cause arthritis of the neck:

- bone cancer: metastasis to the epidural space with progressive onset, producing radicular (spinal nerve root) pain and minimal other signs
- metastasizing tumors originating in breast, kidney, thyroid, or lungs
- myeloma: visible on x-ray, causes hypercalcemia with increased alkaline phosphatase.

Cervicobrachial neuralgia

This is frequently a complication of simple cervical pain of arthritic or mechanical origin. Other causes include:

- metastatic cervical cancer
- tuberculosis of the spine (Pott's disease)
- intra-radicular schwannoma (neoplasm originating from Schwann cells)
- cancer or tuberculosis of the larynx

- adenitis (inflammation of glands), tonsillitis, acute lymphadenitis
- sore throat, dental caries, inflammation of cervical nodes and surrounding connective tissues.

Pain

As with all neuralgias, pain is intense and cannot be mistaken for simple cervical pain. There may be muscle cramps, paresthesia, burning sensation, wrenching, a feeling of "being eaten by an animal," and numbness of the fingers.

The pain is due to the pinching of a nerve root and periradicular venolymphatic congestion, and is relieved by placing the hand behind the head. This relaxes the pressure on the nerve root by improving venolymphatic circulation.

Note: Cervicobrachial neuralgia of mechanical origin does not produce fever, lateral cervical, supraclavicular, or axillary node enlargement, paralysis, abnormal pupil size, facial pain, or sensory deficits.

Temporal arteritis may initially produce occipital/cervical radiating pain that is associated with facial pain.

Vestibular System and Equilibrium

As explained in Chapter 3, trauma to the skull sometimes damages the vestibular sensory system, causing numerous problems with equilibrium and proprioception.

Function of the vestibular system

Essentially, the vestibular system informs the brain about all changes in the body's position.

- It counteracts the force of gravity by coordinating all the required muscular activities and adjustments.
- It regulates the position of the head, torso, and extremities by compensating for and bringing into harmony the forces of acceleration, deceleration, and other forces exerted upon the body.

The vestibular sensory organs convert forces from acceleration of the head or effects of gravity into biological signals. Cerebral control centers use these signals to inform the individual about the orientation of the head, trigger motor reflexes, maintain equilibrium, and coordinate motor functions.

The vestibular sensory organs are activated by movements of the head. Since the force on the organs is equal to their mass times acceleration, and the mass is constant, the force produces biological signals proportional to the acceleration. The CNS processes these signals and activates appropriate motor pathways to keep the head positioned correctly.

The actual receptors for vestibular acceleration are found in the membranous labyrinth of the inner ear, within liquid-filled cavities and canals. The membranous labyrinth is enclosed and protected by the bony labyrinth, inside the petrous portion of the temporal bone.

The vestibular system consists of five sensory units: macula sacculi and macula utriculi (which react to linear acceleration), and ampullary crests of the three semicircular canals (which react to angular acceleration).

Equilibrium function of the vestibular system

Maintenance of equilibrium is a complex process. In addition to the five sensory units of the vestibular system mentioned above, the brain uses information from many other sources, for example, signals from the visual and auditory systems, and from cutaneous, visceral, and osteoarticular mechanoreceptors.

The vestibular sensory organs transform the forces created by acceleration of the head and by gravity into biological signals. One can view the ampullary crests of the semicircular canals as *kinetic receptors*, and the macula utriculi and macula sacculi as *static receptors*.

Vestibular reflexes

These fall into three categories:

- adaptation to changes in direction of gravity—reflexes originating from the maculae
- contraction and coordination of ocular muscles keeping the eyes in the same position during movements—reflexes from the circular canals or otolithic organs
- maintaining posture and muscle tone—reflexes from the ampullary crests and the maculae.

Ciliated cells

For the purpose of maintaining stability, the brain receives innumerable sensory stimuli from the body. All the information coming from the body's mechanoreceptors, the ampulla of the semicircular canals and otoliths, the visual system, and so forth, are instantly processed to give immediate, active motor responses.

Both the semicircular canals and the matrices of the otolithic organs contain ciliated cells. These cells are the point of departure for information received by the vestibular sensory organs and the cochlea. In the cochlea, the ciliated cells are sensitive to sound vibrations. In the vestibular organs, they react to forces of linear and angular acceleration.

Function of ciliated cells

The vestibular system reacts unconsciously and automatically to numerous stimuli. The ciliated cells react primarily to forces created by inertia, when the body is in movement. The force of inertia results in mobilization of the cupulae and otolithic crystals, which send information directly to the ciliated cells. The ciliated cells produce electric signals continuously as the body moves, whether one is consciously aware of the movement or not. An upright body is never completely immobile.

The ciliated cells gather all information from the sensory organs of the inner ear, and their electrical signals increase or diminish depending on the movements and inclination of the head, and intensity of perceived sound.

Proprioceptive and postural systems

All the muscular and tendinous mechanoreceptors play an important role in proprioception. More than 40% of the sensors relaying proprioceptive information are found in the cervical region (Oosterveld, 1991). This helps explain why episodes of vertigo and loss of balance are common in whiplash patients.

Receptors of the proprioceptive system include the vestibular, baroreceptor, plantar, and oculomotor. Joints such as the suboccipital, lumbosacral, and tibiotarsal also contain important receptors.

The sophisticated postural system, under vestibular control, maintains the individual's sense of balance, including control of static equilibrium through muscle tone. This system processes information from the vestibular and proprioceptive systems and many other sources. Vestibular nuclei seem to be activated primarily by oculomotor and nuchal input. The postural system is so complex that most of its connections are still unknown.

Effects of craniocervical trauma on the vestibular system

Acceleration and deceleration forces following collision activate in a violent and intense way the ciliated cells of the semicircular canals and the matrices of the otolithic organs.

When the trauma is violent, some ciliated cells may be partially destroyed. More commonly, they are stunned to the point of no longer transforming body movements into electric signals. In some cases, they become hyper-reactive and generate too many signals, such that the over-stimulated cerebellum can no longer provide reliable information to the body.

PROPRIOCEPTIVE DISINFORMATION SYNDROME

In cases such as the above, the brain receives faulty proprioceptive information and no longer gives appropriate orders to the body. Anti-gravitational muscle function, muscle tone, and posture are not properly maintained.

Because of incorrect activation and poor responses from the cerebellum, the patient has numerous symptoms found also in postural syndrome: loss of balance, vertigo, nausea, motion sickness, poor depth perception, headaches, vertebral pain, and poor visual accommodation.

Proprioceptive disinformation syndrome arises from a variety of cranial and vertebral traumas, for example, sequelae of surgery, dental articulation problems, vertebral arthrosis, sequelae of foot fractures or sprains, and falls on the coccyx.

Post-traumatic Syndromes (Traumatic Neurasthenia)

The possttraumatic syndrome is a well-know clinical complex caused by injury, usually to the head, characterized by neurasthenia, among other symptoms. "Neurasthenia" is a useful, if not very well-defined term. It refers to a syndrome of chronic mental and physical weakness and fatigue, caused by exhaustion of the nervous system. Post-traumatic syndromes occur when the body has received a strong, violent blow, either direct or indirect. The intensity associated with the speed of the blow is the determining factor. Following whiplash or other trauma involving severe, sudden acceleration or deceleration, the victim loses consciousness because of the shock to the brain.

Intense pain may result in fainting. Some falls on the coccyx, for example, because of the pain they cause, trigger a "short circuit" of the nervous system, resulting in a brief fainting spell.

Pathophysiology

Mechanical. The post-traumatic syndrome is due to the blow to the brain within the cranium and to the shock waves transmitted to the different structures of the brain. There may be lesions due to stretching or small tears of dura mater, deformation of neuronal membranes, neuronal ruptures, or destruction of cerebral parenchyma.

Circulatory. Edema following the trauma may impair cerebral circulation. The shock waves can directly or indirectly cause arterial spasms or micro-hemorrhages.

Electrical. Edema always has the potential to create abnormalities in electrical conduction in the brain, for example, coma or cardiac dysrhythmia immediately following impact. Electrical abnormalities of the brain may last a long time, are often not recognized, and can be ameliorated by craniosacral techniques.

Nervous. Dysfunction of certain nerves and nerve centers can produce lasting cerebral or cerebellar vasoconstriction.

Hormonal/chemical. Following trauma, there is an increase of neurotransmitter activity and secretion of catecholamines, kinins, arachidonic acid, serotonin, and histamine.

Psycho-emotional. We believe that some individual cells have a sort of emotional "memory" that can store stresses engendered by trauma.

Cranial post-traumatic syndrome

Here is a partial list of symptoms of cranial post-traumatic syndrome: headache, loss of balance, vertigo, instability, attention deficit, loss of memory or poor memory, asthenia, poor sense of time, insomnia, photophobia, phonophobia, diminished or hightened auditory sensitivity, anosmia or acute sensitivity to smells, emotional instability, behavioral disturbances, depression, neurosis, nausea, diffuse disturbances of the autonomic nervous system, poor adjustment to changes in temperature, sweating, and skin and capillary changes.

Many of these symptoms are difficult to document, and are ignored by insurance companies and managed care plans. These patients have their lives turned upside down, and they drag themselves from one consultant to another. They know that they have genuine internal dysfunction, but standard medical exams do not reveal it.

In such cases, "objective" examinations may be negative—but how well do they represent the more than 100 million neurons which make up the brain? The neurons suffer membranous fractures, and the brain may undergo partial hypoxia or anoxia, which are difficult to document or locate.

Cervical post-traumatic syndrome

This is the source of many consultations following minor or major impacts, often called "whiplash" by the patient. The lesions result from acceleration/deceleration, and hyperextension/hyperflexion of the spinal column. They are accompanied by movements of the cerebral mass, costal, sternal, clavicular, and pleuromediastinal compression or stretching, and movements of certain visceral organs.

Sometimes there is direct trauma to the vertebral artery, resulting in posterior inferior cerebellar artery syndrome (discussed later in this chapter).

The accident victim has sensations of wrenching, internal straining, or deep intense heat in the nape of the neck, which may extend up to the cranium or down to the spine, thorax, or abdomen.

Immediate complaints

Immediately after the injury, the patient does not feel any pain because he is in a desensitized state due to psychological shock and hormonal/chemical reactions. Complaints of pain do not appear until a few days later. We strongly advise against intervention at the early stage. The patient may believe that complaints that appear were caused by your manipulations. Advise him about probable results of the trauma; if you must treat them, use only functional techniques.

Delayed complaints

The most important of these are: cervical pain, upper back pain, headache, cervicobrachial neuralgia, asthenia, depression, vertigo, disturbances of sight or hearing, heaviness of eyelids, paresthesia, and sometimes paresis. Cervical arthrosis may appear years later, concentrated around C4-C5-C6, with osteophytic proliferation on cervical ligaments.

Cervicobrachial neuralgia

This condition is painful and disabling, because of a number of factors:

- *irritation of posterior nerve roots,* through interapophyseal mechanical stress, ligamentous inflammation due to edema, and slight periradicular ischemia
- *strain of the cervicobrachial plexus,* with radicular elongation and tightness at the cervical level. The tightness creates a radicular ischemia, with paresthesia and sometimes paresis.
- *disco-radicular interaction* at the level of the foramen or medullary canal. Protrusion of the disk decreases the size of the medullary canal, and sometimes produces paresis in a distribution which does not seem logical. We have seen patients with complaints of the lower extremity and paresis of the big toe flexor, without any confirmed vertebral lesion. Other patients have significant narrowing of the canals, confirmed by MRI, without any pain.
- *osteoligamentous lesion,* in which the ligaments are strained, stretched, or sometimes torn (microruptures or longitudinal tears). Mechanoreceptors in the ligaments are either stunned or inert, and cannot function properly as sources of information for the local and central nervous systems. They send too many conflicting messages, leading to muscular spasms and vasomotor disturbances.
- *irritation of the cervical sympathetic nervous system* due to interactions between the cervical spine, disks, and nerve roots can create significant intracanal pressure. The inferior cervical ganglion may have a direct or indirect lesion, in which case there is almost always ipsilateral miosis (contraction of the pupil). All lesions in the sympathetic nervous system may bring on parasympathetic problems. The two systems are interdependent, as evidenced by the numerous anastomoses between them. This may explain certain paradoxical post-traumatic reactions.
- *stretching of the cervical dura mater,* with certain nerve roots selectively irritated by their perineuria
- *stretching of the cervicobrachial plexus,* due to an abrupt movement of the spine with respect to an upper extremity, or vice versa. Stretching can result in paresis if severe, or in cervicobrachial neuralgia with associated paresthesia if less severe.

- *stretching of the vertebral artery.* Cervical strain may be associated with restrictions of the vertebral artery at the C5-C6 or C1-C2 levels. Vaso-constriction of this artery can reduce or stop its blood flow, with resulting cere-bellar problems.

Post-traumatic tearing of the vertebral artery

The wall of the vertebral artery may be injured by trauma, typically between C1 and C2. Damage to the tunica intima produces an arterial thrombosis, or, less frequently, arterial or venous fistulas.

Symptomatology

Symptoms appear either very soon or not until two or three weeks after the trauma! It is useless, and potentially dangerous, to manipulate the spinal column in the days immediately following trauma.

The symptoms of vertebral artery tearing include: cervical pain, cervicobrachial neuralgia, occipitofrontal headache, brief positional and rotatory vertigo, problems with hearing and vision, drop attacks, paresthesia, paresis, cranial nerve dysfunction (diplopia, hypoesthesia, facial paresis, problems with swallowing and vocalization), neurasthenia, and depression.

Predisposing factors

The primary predisposing factors for tearing are hypoplasia or agenesis of the ver-tebral artery, and problems with the thoracic outlet. Dysplasias of the artery range from simple folding to fibromuscular lesions involving its entire course.

Upper cervical syndrome

Above the level of C4, the spine may suffer from twisting and rotating motions, especially at the level of C1-C2. These movements may rupture the vertebral artery at the level of C2, irritate the cervical sympathetic nervous plexus, or stretch the dura mater.

Inferior cervical syndrome

This syndrome occurs when vertebral artery tearing is below the level of C4. In theory, the artery is protected by the wide amplitude of flexion and extension of the spine. However, it may be irritated and suffer vasomotor problems in lateral cervicotho-racic shocks which irritate the stellar ganglion. Soft intervertebral disk hernias are found most frequently between C5/C6.

Post-traumatic cervical arthrosis

We believe that this occurs inevitably after trauma involving the spine, and may persist for years. Sometimes symptoms don't appear until decades later!

Pathophysiology

The cartilaginous system and joints are violently stretched. Because of the speed of the trauma, the muscles cannot respond effectively to protect the spine. Irritation of the cartilage leads to inflammation, consequent stimulation of chondrocytes, and eventual ossification affecting the ligaments.

We are amazed by how often medical practitioners declare that arthrosis causes cervical restriction, when actually the reverse is true. Likewise, the well-known "lipping" seen on x-rays is really the manifestation and not the cause of abnormal mechanical articular tension.

Nerve disorders

There are numerous disorders created by compression of the cervicobrachial plexus which produce neuralgia, paresthesia, and (thankfully, more rarely) paresis of the upper extremities. These disorders may affect the thorax or lower extremities.

Vascular disorders

Intracanal and intratransversal narrowing may produce, through reflex or direct mechanical compression, a decrease of vertebrobasilar output. Extrinsic compression is most often found between C4/C6, while osteophytes push the vertebral artery back.

Reduced output of the vertebral artery is rarely due to direct mechanical compression from osteophytic and intertransversal proliferation. We believe that irritation of the sympathetic nervous system creates vasoconstriction of the vertebral artery. The lower part, where the artery begins near the inferior cervical ganglion, is the most involved.

With osteophytic compression of the canal, even a slight blow or muscular/ligamentous pressure can disrupt arterial flow. There is a system of reciprocal compensation between the two vertebral arteries. When only one side is affected, the other tends to compensate. When both sides are affected, symptoms are more severe and treatment is difficult.

Cervicocephalic syndrome

This syndrome is usually due to intracanal or intratransversal narrowing, produced by arthrosis of the cervical spine. Principal symptoms are described below.

Vertigo

This occurs most often in women between 35 and 50 years of age, and may be aggravated by circulatory dysfunctions due to menopause. Vertigo is positional, intense, and of short duration. It occurs when the head is rotated or extended with the arms in the air, in the transition from lying down to standing, or vice versa.

The patient, fearful of triggering vertigo, takes precautionary measures such as turning the whole body rather than just the head in order to see. To reduce anxiety, it is important to explain to the patient the cause of her vertigo, and sensible precautions for avoiding it.

Headaches

Headaches associated with this syndrome are occipitofrontal, retro-orbital, diffuse, bilateral, and continuous with a few paroxysmal outbursts. They often originate in the suboccipital region. This distinguishes them from migraines and other headaches arising from digestive, hormonal, or psychological causes, which almost always begin in the frontal or anterior parietal region.

Auditory disturbances

These include ringing in the ears, tinnitus, a sensation that the ears are clogged, earache, and ringing produced or accentuated by movements of the neck. The ringing may be either continuous or pulsatile, as if the patient feels a pinched arteriole in the depths of the ear.

Visual disturbances

These include rapid tiring of the eyes when reading or watching movies or television, blurred vision, burning eyes, scotoma, flickering, eye pain, photophobia, blepharospasm, and diploplia.

Disturbances of taste and smell

We have seen about a dozen patients who have lost the sense of smell, either partially or totally, after trauma. Results from our treatment of these patients have been somewhat disappointing.

Paresthesias

These are pharyngeal dysesthesias and vasomotor seizures of the face, sometimes accompanied by problems with phonation. Long automobile trips and activities in which the spine is strained may bring about cervical pain, paresthesias, or, less frequently, facial vasomotor disturbances.

Neck pain

This is common, but remains in the background. It may be accompanied by painful cervicobrachial neuralgia during certain movements, especially at night.

The patient presents with unilateral radiating pain, caused by foraminal narrowing of osteophytic origin. Radicular pain fluctuates between very sharp and dull. There may be a unilateral burning of the scalp, or sensitivity when combing the hair.

Digestive signs

Intracanal or foraminal osteophytic compression, when those structures are subjected to repeated mechanical stress, produces digestive problems of the hepatobiliary or (much less frequently) gastric region. In our experience, restrictions on the left are more often accompanied by bowel problems, while those on the right typically involve the liver.

Cardiac signs

Left cervical restrictions may produce precordialgias and problems of cardiac rhythm, and are often accompanied by restriction of the fourth left costovertebral joint. We believe, without definitive proof, that they sometimes produce coronary vasoconstriction.

Reflex Sympathetic Dystrophy

One possible consequence of trauma is the development of reflex sympathetic dystrophy (RSD). This is a complex and poorly understood phenomenon, as reflected by the alternative names given to it, for example, algodystrophy, causalgia. Because the relation of this syndrome to the autonomic nervous system is not totally clear, some authors prefer to use the term complex regional pain syndrome (CRPS) instead of RSD.

Definition

RSD is a collection of polymorphic pathologic signs in conjunction with vasomotor and sudomotor disturbances, triggered by trauma and a variety of stresses. Predisposing factors are disturbances of the autonomic nervous system, metabolic disturbances (hypertriglyceridemia, diabetes), and psychological disturbances (depression, anxiety).

Pain is of the inflammatory or mechanical type. There are notable pseudo-inflammatory effects, of varying intensity, which may involve one or more articular regions and affect various tissue layers, from the skin to the bone.

Etiology

There has been much controversy about the etiology of RSD, but it appears to be related to trauma-induced dysfunction of the autonomic nervous system. Its diagnosis can also be controversial. While simple for typical cases, diagnosis can be quite difficult for atypical or monosymptomatic cases, especially in the absence of the decalcification changes apparent on x-ray—which may take many months to be manifested.

RSD is very common. Many atypical or incomplete forms escape detection. In perhaps 50% of cases, there is no obvious etiologic factor. In the other 50%, RSD is associated with trauma, surgical procedures, immobility from a cast, or various nontraumatic conditions, including:

- peripheral or central nervous system dysfunction
- cardiovascular disorders
- pleuropulmonary disorders
- endocrine disorders
- benign tumors
- malignant tumors (primary or secondary)
- pregnancy
- medications (especially barbiturates and antitubercular medications).

Regardless of severity, trauma is the cause of around 70% of RSD in the lower extremities, and 40% in the upper extremities.

Clinical progression

Warming phase

The first phase of RSD usually has a gradual onset and is marked by intermittent or constant pain of variable intensity, triggered by movement or by weight-bearing. There is usually a localized increase in warmth, and some functional loss of mobility, which can be severe. The appearance of the affected region is either normal or inflamed, with reddening of the skin, cutaneous hyperthermia, and hyperesthesia. This phase may be short, or even go unnoticed, but it can also last for weeks or months

Cooling phase

The later phase of RSD is marked by generalized cooling. The pain may persist, but with an intermittent quality. The functional loss of mobility may remain. The appearance of the affected area is either normal, edematous, or erythrocyanotic, especially toward the periphery. Outright hypothermia has replaced hyperthermia. Atrophy of the subcutaneous tissue and interstitial muscle occurs. There can also be thickening of joint capsules, stiffness with flexion deformity of the fingers, induration of the skin, and features reminiscent of scleroderma.

Finally, there are trophic changes and contracture of the skin and joints, with radiographic evidence of severe demineralization in the painful areas. This may be associated with fibrosis, retraction of tendons, capsules, and aponeuroses, and gross restriction of movement.

Biochemistry

At the biochemical level, there are no signs characteristic of RSD. Inflammatory signs are absent and sedimentation rate is normal. In cases of joint effusion, the synovial fluid is of the mechanical type. One often finds calcemia, calciuria, phosphoremia, alkaline phosphates, and elevated hydroxyprolinuria.

Imaging studies

Radioimaging signs which provide the conventional basis for diagnosis of RSD are inconsistent and appear late. Their appearance, intensity, topography, and reproducibility vary considerably from one individual to the next. X-ray films must be of high quality, and include both the affected and non-affected side for comparison, as well as other joints. Radiological abnormalities suggestive of RSD appear several weeks to months after the initial functional signs. Typical x-rays of RSD show demineralization of variable intensity, mostly in the subchondral regions. There may be some compression of vertebrae; otherwise, there is no deformation of the bones or pathological fracture, despite the prevalence of demineralization.

Bone scan reveals premature hyperfixation, usually intense and sometimes intermittent. This may appear at the beginning of the functional signs, but persists longer, and usually regresses before other radiological signs do.

CAT scan is of limited use for diagnosis of RSD. MRI, mainly at the level of the hip, allows differential diagnosis of osteonecrosis versus RSD.

Manual thermal diagnosis

The affected areas initially radiate heat and are easy to detect. After a variable period of time, hypothermia replaces the hyperthermia, as explained above.

Clinical variation

There are numerous variations on the typical pattern. Incomplete forms with isolated soft tissue changes may be restricted to just the joint capsules, tendons, aponeuroses, or synovial membranes. Other attenuated forms present as tendinitis, capsulitis, arthrosis, or tenosynovitis. Forms resembling rheumatoid disease occur bilaterally in the upper extremities. Sometimes a partial or fragmented form can complicate the diagnosis, for example, only one finger of one hand, or part of a femoral condyle.

The manifestation of RSD varies, depending on which part of the body is involved.

- RSD of the hand, in its most common form, is easy to recognize. A few weeks after trauma, which may have healed and been forgotten, pain appears (over the course of a few hours or days) with swelling of the wrist and the whole hand. The fingers become stiff, half-flexed, and swollen, and any attempt to move them causes sharp pain. The skin is smooth, pink or red, and hot to the touch.
- The hand and shoulder may both be affected. This is the classic "shoulder-hand" syndrome which may follow trauma to the upper extremity *or a myocardial infarct*. Besides pain in the shoulder, there is capsular retraction with restriction of passive mobility, especially in abduction and lateral rotation. Symptoms may be limited to the shoulder. It is rare for the elbow to be affected.
- In the lower extremity, the foot is the part most frequently affected by RSD, usually as a result of trauma. The onset may be sudden, presenting as an episode of gout. The pain and edema of the foot and ankle make walking difficult. The hip undergoes functional loss of mobility, with a normal or subnormal passive mobility. This may occur in late pregnancy or after delivery. The knee is rarely affected; when it is, the symptoms mimic arthritis or arthrosis.
- When the spine is affected by a late post-traumatic collapse of a vertebral body, also known as Kümmell's spondylitis, there is sharp pain in the spine which mimics cervical pain, back pain, or acute lumbalgia. When the anterior thoracic wall is affected, it may be the original site or secondary to a myocardial infarction.

Some RSDs have symptoms which are continuous; others occur in repeated episodes.

Differential diagnosis

Differential diagnosis can be difficult, especially in the atypical or incomplete forms. Furthermore, other disorders which may be confused with RSD sometimes cause an attack of actual RSD.

- Arthritis (inflammatory, septic, gouty, or tubercular) has an associated increase in sedimentation rate, hyperleucocytosis, and inflammatory or purulent synovial liquid.
- Septic tenosynovitis (phlegmons of the tendinous sheath) is associated with hyperleucocytosis and increased sedimentation rate.
- Infection and dislocation of joint prosthesis, which are not always seen on x-ray.
- Benign tumors such as osteoid osteoma are difficult to diagnose. Night time worsening of pain, and dramatic effectiveness of aspirin and non-steroidal anti-inflammatory drugs, suggest osteoid osteoma.
- Malignant tumors, primary or secondary, require a bone biopsy.

- Aseptic osteonecrosis of the head or condyle of a femur.
- Arthrosis
- Fatigue fractures present a pseudo-inflammatory picture similar to arthrosis. In both cases, x-ray is normal in the beginning.
- Sprains are often difficult to differentiate from spontaneous RSD when the patient believes he has suffered a sprain.
- Tendonitis is difficult to distinguish when RSD presents as an isolated tendon being affected.
- Somatic conversion disorder is difficult to distinguish from RSD in cases of isolated pain without or before any changes on x-ray. Bone scan is normal in conversion disorder.

Pathophysiology

Many previous theories on the nature of RSD (infectious, endocrine, inflammatory) have been abandoned. Since the work of Leriche and Sudeck in the earlier 1900s (for review see Doury, 1984), it is accepted that the pathologic signs grouped under RSD result from vasomotor disturbances (primarily vascular stasis) brought on by a variety of stresses. These stresses, sometimes very ordinary ones, give rise to nociceptive reactions, which in turn trigger afferent impulses responsible for the vasomotor disturbances. These phenomena occur through a reflex arc with sensory nerves acting as the afferent pathway, the autonomic formations of the spinal cord in the middle, and postganglionic sympathetic fibers as the efferent pathway. Higher CNS centers which regulate vasomotor functions, and certain neurotransmitters (e.g., serotonin) may also be involved.

Principles of treatment

It is rare that patients come to see us for RSD alone. However, we note mild signs of it in many patients who come to us after trauma. It is important to take the RSD into account in treating such patients.

Medications may be helpful during the acute phase, but it is essential to let the affected region rest. We must admit that osteopathic treatment cannot resolve all the effects of RSD, although we have sometimes been able to bring relief.

Osteopathic treatment must be the gentlest possible, at a distance from the inflammatory lesions, and employing mechanical manipulation which is *the least traumatic*. There are several levels of tissue affected simultaneously, and one within the other, like Russian dolls.

Movement of the joints in the affected area is proscribed if this triggers or increases pain. The principle of *"Primum non nocere"* (first, cause no pain) should always guide osteopathic treatment. Any nociceptive overload will simply aggravate the inflammatory process and counteract the desired result. The objective is to reduce vascular stasis, acting either directly on mechanical obstacles or indirectly via the autonomic system, in order to increase vascular output.

To effectively treat RSD, you must check and free the anatomic components of the autonomic pathway, especially the plexus and cord segments involved. You can also produce an effect on the neuro-endocrine regulatory system via the primary respiratory mechanism.

Vertebrobasilar Insufficiency

We see a surprisingly high number of cases of vertebrobasilar system disorder. Often the condition has existed for a number of years, and the patient is accustomed to the symptoms and doesn't believe there is a remedy. These patients lead cautious lives, avoiding positions with the arms raised or neck extended, and rapid changes in position.

Vertebrobasilar artery system

This system supplies much of the posterior neck and brain. It is a vital component for proper circulation of the head *(Fig. 4-1)*.

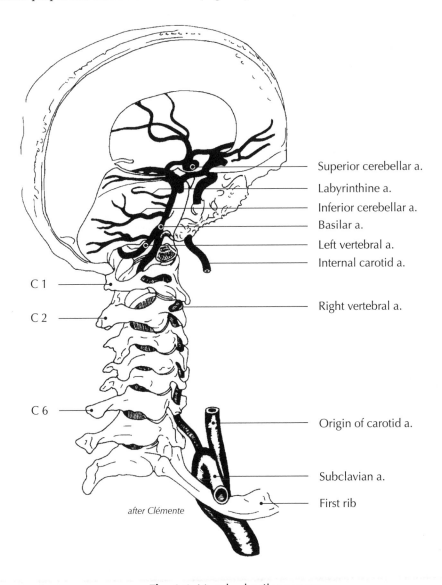

Superior cerebellar a.

Labyrinthine a.

Inferior cerebellar a.

Basilar a.

Left vertebral a.

Internal carotid a.

Right vertebral a.

C 1

C 2

C 6

Origin of carotid a.

Subclavian a.

First rib

after Clémente

Fig. 4-1: Vertebrobasilar system

Vertebral artery

This occupies most of the transverse canal. It is accompanied by a plexus of veins surrounded by sympathetic fibers. The latter, when irritated, may cause vasoconstriction, which in turn produces numerous functional problems.

Basilar artery

The two vertebral arteries unite to form the basilar trunk, 4-5mm in diameter and 2.5 to 4.5cm long. The basilar artery ends in the interpeduncular space, where it divides into the two posterior cerebral arteries which supply the posterior part of the brain, occipital lobes, hypothalamus, and part of the mesencephalon. The intracranial collaterals of the vertebral arteries and the basilar trunk supply the upper cervical spinal cord, part of the medulla, cerebral trunk, part of the cerebellum, and inner ear *(Fig. 4-2)*.

Vertebrobasilar system

The vertebral arteries are heavily anastomosed, with the largest anastomosis at the level of the basilar trunk. They are linked by the anterior spinal artery and the medullary branches, and are connected to certain branches of the external carotid and subclavian arteries.

Positional variations in output, and compensation mechanisms

In view of the importance of the areas supplied by the vertebrobasilar system, it is easy to see how serious and pathogenic variations in blood flow can be. The body must have mechanisms to completely compensate for such variation, and adequate blood supply to the cerebrum and cerebellum.

During rotation of the neck, the output of the vertebral artery on the side opposite the rotation is reduced. At maximal rotation, carotid output is also diminished. *Rotation combined with extension of the neck reduces output of the contralateral vertebral artery by ~30%*. Normally, this creates automatic circulatory compensation by the ipsilateral vertebral artery. Such compensation is easily accomplished in a subject who has no trauma or arthrosis. It is much more difficult in a patient with cervical arthrosis and abnormal muscular/ligamentous tension.

We repeat our warning to avoid cervical manipulations with the cervical spine extended and rotated. In this position, vertebral artery output is diminished, and the artery is stretched in its inter-transversal course below C2, and in its bends around the occipital/atlas/axis.

Stretching of the sympathetic nerve plexus triggers a vasoconstriction reflex, which further diminishes vertebral artery output and consequently basilar circulation. *We have been able to prove, using the Doppler effect, an increase in vertebrobasilar output of between 25 to 30%* after freeing certain joints of the thoracic passage and mobilizing the back. We have wondered for a long time whether this increase is of reflex or hormonal/chemical origin. The speed of the change suggests a reflex triggered by local mechanoreceptors.

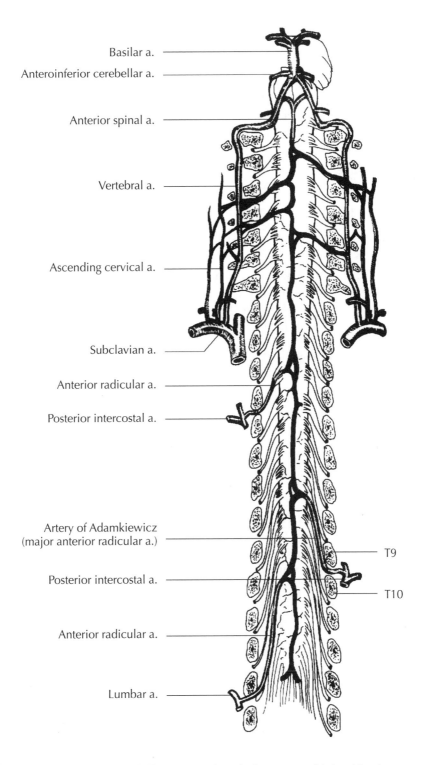

Basilar a.

Anteroinferior cerebellar a.

Anterior spinal a.

Vertebral a.

Ascending cervical a.

Subclavian a.

Anterior radicular a.

Posterior intercostal a.

Artery of Adamkiewicz
(major anterior radicular a.)

Posterior intercostal a.

Anterior radicular a.

Lumbar a.

T9

T10

Fig. 4-2: Arterial medullary network with the artery of Adamkiewicz
(posterior view of an open column)

Mechanical compressions

Arthrosis

Arthrosis of the vertebrae or disk, and inflammation of the interapophyseal joints, affect the vertebral artery. The artery may actually be pushed back by boney proliferation. In such cases, diminished output occurs on the side of the rotation.

Other mechanical compressions

These include:

- malformations of the occipitocervical junction (e.g., in the basilar impression)
- fibrosis and inflammation of the joints of the scalene muscle
- lower cervical bone spurs
- costoclavicular torsion
- various tumors
- sequelae of cervicothoracic trauma
- pleuropulmonary sequelae
- fusion of the first costovertebral joint
- costoclavicular boney calluses.

Indirect action of arthrosis

In arthrosis of the cervical spine, the vertebral nerves may be mechanically irritated and produce vasoconstriction of the artery. Boney proliferation, affecting the vertebral canal, may also cause reflex vasoconstriction of the vertebral artery.

Reflex effect

Any disorder of the cervical sympathetic chain, or vertebral fusion, may affect the size of the vertebral artery. Numerous tissue restrictions, of muscular/ligamentous or visceral origin, can have a reflex effect on the arterial wall.

Vertebral vein

Output of the vein cannot vary in response to reflex spasm, as is the case with the neighboring artery. The vein requires a thoracic inspiratory space for efficient circulation. Anything that hinders the transmission of negative intravenous pressure affects the vertebral vein. Problems of the cervicothoracic junction frequently affect vertebral vein circulation.

Cushing phenomenon

In this phenomenon, intracranial pressure rises acutely, usually to more than 50% of systolic arterial pressure. This is related to changes in the vascular system. Intrathoracic pressures have a direct effect on drainage of veins in the head and neck, including the jugular veins and vertebral veins.

A study lead by Swierzewski (1994) found that about 37% of cranial trauma has associated thoracic trauma. It is therefore important to free the muscular/ligamentous and fascial systems of the thoracic outlet in order to improve venous and lymph circulation of the cranium.

We believe that restrictions of the kidney also play an important reactive role in vertebrobasilar circulation.

Other etiologies of vertebrobasilar insufficiency

- atheromatosis, implicated in the formation of atheroma, arterial hypertension, tobacco addiction, diabetes, oral contraceptives, and certain forms of trauma. These can split, detach, and cause plaques of atheroma to migrate.

- atherosclerosis, found mostly in the ostium of the vertebral or subclavian artery
- stenosis or thrombosis of the subclavian artery, leading to circulatory diversion
- dysplasia which shows a "string of pearls" picture
- forceful manipulation of the spinal column in extension/rotation may cause intimal tearing or arterial thrombosis
- tearing of blood vessel walls
- emboli

Symptoms of vertebrobasilar insufficiency

These reflect inadequate blood flow to specific areas, namely, the upper cervical spinal cord, medulla, cerebrum, cerebellum, and/or inner ear. Symptoms include:

- vestibular syndrome with positional vertigo
- ophthalmic signs: blurred vision, loss of color vision, reduced acuity, visual hallucinations
- oculomotor problems: paresis, drop attacks (falling on one's knees without loss of consciousness or vertigo) of short duration triggered by rotation of the head
- headaches of medium intensity, beginning at the suboccipital level and radiating toward the front
- paresthesia of the arms, hands, lower body, or one side of the face
- cerebellar disorders: instability, loss of equilibrium
- tinnitus, affecting cranial nerve VIII
- hypoacusis or hyperacusis (reduced or acute acoustic sensitivity): the branch of the basilar artery to the inner ear is involved in problems with auditory acuity
- problems with sleeping, alertness, and memory.

Thoracic Outlet Syndrome

The thoracic outlet is often the site of mechanical problems which impact lymphatic, arterial, and venous circulation of the head, neck, and thorax. It has several structural components, described below.

Costoscalene passage

This is delimited inferiorly by the first rib, anteriorly by the anterior scalene, and posteriorly by the middle scalene. Compression of this passage has vascular and nervous consequences, because the primary arteries of the cervicobrachial plexus are right behind the vascular structures which pass near the scalenes.

Costoclavicular passage

This is defined superiorly by the subclavian muscle, its aponeurosis, and the internal surface of the clavicle. Inferiorly, it is delimited by the upper surface of the first rib, anterior scalene tendon, and middle cervical aponeurosis.

Large movements of the shoulder normally produce a physiological compression of the costoclavicular passage. Muscular or ligamentous problems may cause rapid compression of arteries, veins, and lymph vessels in this area.

Subpectoral tunnel

The vascular nerve passes underneath the tendon of the pectoralis minor, near its coracoid insertion. The coracoclavicular ligaments permit the pectoralis minor to play a role in compression. In reality this subpectoral compression is rare, because the pectoralis minor acts indirectly on the coracoid and its ligaments to create or to increase costoclavicular compression.

Compression of the thoracic outlet

The major anatomical elements in this region are naturally compressed, not only by the large movements of the shoulder (depression and retraction of the scapula, abduction and lateral rotation of the arm), but also by rotation and extension of the spine.

People with a muscular/ligamentous problem in this area may suffer vascular nerve problems just from carrying a bag with a strap across the chest, or even wearing a seat belt. (*The Lancet* [346:1044, 1995] reports an incident of fainting when the driver turned to the right while wearing a seat belt! The carotid sinus was hypersensitive to mechanical compression by turning the head.)

Etiology

Thoracic outlet syndrome has many possible causes. We can divide them into three categories.

Boney structures

- apophysitis of C7, less frequently C6
- cervical rib, or agenesis of the first rib (replaced by fibrous tissue)
- subclavicular or subcostal boney callus, post-fracture
- costoclavicular misalignment of congenital or fetal malpositional origin. This condition is often overlooked. However, we believe that it is common, and conducive to costothoracic outlet compression.
- scoliosis
- deforming osteofibrous sequelae of cervicothoracic trauma

Soft tissue structures

- unusual insertion of anterior scalene muscle
- double insertion of middle scalene muscle
- fibromuscular retractions in the costoclavicular or costovertebral regions
- costovertebral C7/T1 fusion
- sternoclavicular and acromioclavicular restrictions
- cervicopleural restrictions, secondary to infection or trauma

- asthenic habitus and general iatrogenic hypotonias (anxiolytics, antidepressants, barbiturates)

Circulatory/ general causes

These include atheromatosis, arteriosclerosis, thromboses, arterial diseases, arterial malformation, anatomical misalignment.

Women are more likely to experience compression of the cervical thoracic outlet because of the greater slant of their clavicles and first ribs.

Symptoms of thoracic outlet syndrome

Paresthesia of upper extremities

The hands are most often affected, the forearms and arms more rarely. Of the vertebrae, C7/T1 are the most often affected. Radiation begins at the medial surface of the arms, continues along the ulnar edge of the forearm, and ends at the ring and little fingers.

Patients try various movements and positions in an attempt to reduce nerve irritation. They often put the affected hand behind the neck in order to find fleeting relief from pain.

Scapulohumeral periarthritis may follow compression of the thoracic outlet, due to compression of a sensitive capsular branch. Less often, one sees short middle costal radiations, precordial in men and to the breasts in women.

Arterial signs

These appear in relationship to body position. After lying too long on the same side, the subject gets out of bed and feels finger cramps with loss of mobility. An important sign is the feeling of numbness in the fingers, which the subject shakes frequently in order to regain some sensation. It is a kind of unilateral Raynaud's disease. The symptoms are most pronounced when the arms are up and the head is extended.

Venous/ lymphatic signs

The subclavian vein, in front of the artery, is the first to be compressed in certain movements or positions. Compensations for this are more effective than for arterial disorders; among our patients with thoracic outlet syndrome, only about 15% present clear venous signs: swollen fingers, bluish skin color, localized sweating.

The symptoms are enhanced by muscular activity. The upper extremities feel heavy, and there is cyanosis and edema of the hand, which improve with rest. With arms raised and head tilted back, the venous/lymphatic symptoms take longer to appear. This position may even improve the symptoms temporarily.

General signs

General signs of thoracic outlet syndrome include: vertigo, headache, nausea, instability, loss of equilibrium, poor spatial sense, slight psychomotor lack of coordination, tinnitus, hyperacusis, memory loss, reduced cognitive capacity, general digestive problems, and superficial thoracoabdominal pain.

Many of these are related to subclavian artery compression, especially on its collateral branch, the vertebral artery. The internal mammary artery is not involved.

Vertigo

One patient in seven goes to a general practitioner because of "vertigo." Like headaches, this is a catch-all category in which simple, benign cases are thrown together with more serious ones.

Vertigo may be accompanied by labyrinthine signs: deafness, tinnitus, feeling of fullness in the ears.

Benign paroxysmal positional vertigo

This may occur when otoliths detach from the ventricular macula, which evaluate linear displacements of the head. This creates an imbalance in utricular activity and displacement of the crystals floating in the endolymphatic spaces. The otoliths settle on the cupula of the posterior semicircular canal and produce an intense rotatory vertigo of brief duration (about 20 seconds) in certain positions of the head. This process modifies the mass of the posterior semicircular canal, thereby enhancing pressure receptivity.

One can provoke this response using Hallpike's maneuver: the patient changes quickly from sitting position to lying down, or vice versa. In the case of benign paroxysmal positional vertigo, the patient experiences a strong rotatory vertigo associated with geotrophic rotational nystagmus on the side of the affected ear, almost always with a delay. (This helps distinguish it from vertigo due to CNS disease, which appears without a delay but is less intense.) The nystagmus often persists and does not reverse when sitting up.

Etiology

Craniocervical trauma promotes this sort of vertigo by causing restrictions in the otolithic membrane. Irritation of the cervical sympathetic nerve and edema of damaged tissues cause a reduction in vertebral artery output and indirect restriction of the otolithic membrane.

Pathogenesis

Following trauma or circulatory problems, changes in labyrinthine fluid pressure lead to lithiasis of the cupula, and consequent formation of otoliths.

Remarks

ENT specialists, in treating these patients, place them in a position to trigger the nystagmus and vertigo, then move them in a seesaw fashion with 180° rotation in order to reverse the position of the cupula so that the otoliths are dispersed. We have achieved good results with some types of vertigo by manipulation—particularly direct vertebral mobilization. We examine the seated patient to determine which level to mobilize, then rapidly place the patient in supine position and perform the manipulation. In some cases, successful outcome may result not from the manipulation, but rather from the simple fact of placing the patient rapidly in a horizontal position, and thereby dispersing the otoliths!

Postural syndrome

This occurs after cervical or cranial trauma, particularly whiplash. It may first appear months or even years after the accident. Common signs include brief vertigo when moving the neck, impression of floating, motion sickness, difficulty with night driving, poor depth perception, headaches, and back pain.

Vertigo of vascular origin

Etiology

This type of vertigo can result from a variety of primary vascular problems secondary to other conditions leading to vascular dysfunction:

- aging and associated atherosclerosis
- emboli, thrombosis
- congenital vascular abnormalities
- acquired arterial disease (aneurysms, diseases of the arterial walls)
- anxiety attacks, depression
- temporo-mandibular dysfunction and dental problems
- osteoarticular, myofascial, ligamentous, or cervical pathology.

Reversible vertigo of vascular origin

This form is repetitive and of short duration, with a favorable prognosis. Principal causes are described in the following sections.

VERTEBROBASILAR INSUFFICIENCY

Vertigo is positional and due to rapid hemodynamic modification. There is a reduction of vertebral artery flow, most often in the cervical section, and sometimes associated with arterial spasm or atheromatous lesions.

TRANSIENT VESTIBULAR ISCHEMIA

Vertigo is the result of transient ischemic attacks affecting the vestibular nuclei. Predisposing conditions are:

- cervical pain, irritating the cervical sympathetic chain and causing spasm of the vertebral artery
- arthrosis of the cervical spine and disks, compressing the vertebral artery
- apophysitis and other congenital malformations
- cervical trauma.

CLINICAL EXAMINATION AND DIAGNOSIS

For a diagnosis of reversible vertigo of vascular origin, a key sign is asymmetrical blood pressure, typically lower pressure on the side with the restriction. Other signs:

- a positive Adson's test on the side with the restriction
- a cervical vascular bruit revealed by auscultation of the neck
- mobility tests reveal cervical or cervicothoracic restrictions.

PATHOPHYSIOLOGY

Movement of the head interrupts flow of one of the vertebral arteries, through either compression of the vertebral foramen, or spasm, or both. Vertigo of vascular origin is of short duration, and hard to differentiate from benign paroxysmal vertigo caused by otoliths.

Central vestibular disorders often occur with vertebrobasilar circulatory insufficiency, as described in Chapter 5 below. In this case, symptoms are reversible and electronystagmography appears normal.

Interestingly, this type of vertigo does not occur when the patient is lying on the stomach. We believe that in this position the otoliths are less mobilized and do not stimulate the labyrinthine centers much, and intracerebral pressure is slightly elevated. Flex the neck as far as possible for about 30 seconds.

In order to keep the patient's trust during examination, it is important not to trigger vertigo by changes of position. If the patient is lying on the back, flex the neck as far as possible for about 30 seconds before letting him get up.

Vertigo from Ménière's disease

Ménière's disease is more common than many practitioners realize. It has been suggested that van Gogh had this disease and that he mutilated himself because of it. Some main signs:

- rotatory vertigo lasting more than 30 minutes but less than 2 hours
- unilateral deafness with a feeling of fullness in the affected ear
- unilateral tinnitis with low pitched overtones (see below)
- sensory deficits without any decrease in reflexes (see below).

PATHOPHYSIOLOGY

The cause of vertigo from Ménière's disease is not completely clear. Some authorities believe it is an idiopathic hydrops (abnormal accumulation of serous fluid) due to insufficient reabsorption of endolymph by the endolymphatic sac, which was affected by autoimmune reaction, or by embryopathic, infectious, genetic, or traumatic causes. Idiopathic hydrops causes increased pressure, dilatation, or distention of the membranous labyrinth.

The membranous labyrinth is bathed in perilymph that separates it from the bony labyrinth. The latter is made up of cavities communicating with each other and forming a closed system filled with endolymph. There are two portions:

- the anterior labyrinth or cochlear canal, the *organ of hearing*
- the posterior labyrinth, including the semicircular canals, utricle, and sacculus—the *organ of equilibrium.*

Pressure increase due to hydrops may raise the pressure of the basilar membrane and compress the acoustic papillae. The increase in fluid volume alters the vibrational qualities of the cochlear canal, leading gradually to deafness. The same process may occur at the vestibular level.

SPECIAL CHARACTERISTICS

The tinnitus has low pitched overtones like a conch shell, with a feeling of a full ear. Hypoacusis, if present, makes the tinnitus sharper. Rotatory vertigo is often intense and accompanied by nausea and vomiting. The attacks can be triggered by many factors, including emotional shock. Sometimes the vertigo is very transient. Unfortunately, the deafness can be irreversible.

There are premenstrual and perimenopausal variations of Ménière's syndrome, as mentioned briefly later. For these, the symptoms often improve spontaneously.

Irreversible vertigo of vascular origin

These patients rarely come to us for consultation during the early stages of this problem, for they are immediately sent to specialists. They have posterior inferior cerebellar artery syndrome (discussed later in this chapter) or thrombosis of the labyrinthine artery. The latter causes ischemia, deafness with areflexia due to necrosis of the labyrinth, and vertigo. The vertigo disappears after a few days because of CNS compensations.

Vertigo from vestibular neuritis

Vestibular neuritis, often of viral origin, affects the vestibular nerve but not the structures of the inner ear. It produces severe vertigo lasting three days, moderate vertigo lasting about three weeks, and minimal vertigo lasting three months. Hearing is not affected, but there is a loss of lateral balance, horizontal rotational nystagmus, nausea, and vomiting.

Vertigo from labyrinthitis

This is an inflammation of the inner ear of viral, bacterial, or toxic origin. Again, severe vertigo lasts for three days, moderate instability for about three weeks, and discomfort for three months. There can be neurosensory auditory effects, for example, Ménière's disease.

Vertigo from acoustic neurinoma

This is not a true vertigo, rather a feeling of instability. It is caused by a schwannoma located in the inferior vestibular section of the vestibulocochlear nerve. There is a unilateral deafness accompanied by a slight instability or feeling of imbalance.

The tumor gradually destroys the fibers of the vestibular nerve, resulting in a vestibular deficit which is compensated by the underlying vestibular nuclei of the cerebral trunk. Other signs are facial hemispasm, unilateral otalgia, headache, and hemianesthesia.

Vertigo from multiple sclerosis

This disease is too difficult to diagnose in the beginning because its symptoms are indistinct and nonspecific: problems of equilibrium, feeling unstable or drunk. A sudden onset of equilibrium problems, which then spontaneously resolve, points toward MS. Other symptoms include paresthesia, rapid decline in visual acuity, diplopia, and a sudden sensation of electric shock in the body when the neck is flexed.

We have seen a case of MS where the only initial symptom was slight itching on the medial surface of the thigh!

One has to look for pyramidal, cerebellar, and sensory signs. Ophthalmoplegia (paralysis of the eye muscles) is responsible for the diplopia, while monocular nystagmus creates an impression of vertigo and shifting of objects.

Vertigo from central vestibular syndrome

This condition is a result of lesions in the CNS connections between vestibular nuclei, usually due to modification or diversion of vertebrobasilar blood flow following atheroma, congenital abnormalities, or mechanical problems. There are basically two types: a central vestibular syndrome with instability, and a peripheral vestibular syndrome with rotatory vertigo and many disturbances of the autonomic nervous system. Signs vary in intensity, and may appear singly or in combinations. We seldom see cases of vestibular syndrome since they are usually referred to ENT specialists or a hospital.

Proprioceptive and other pathways governing equilibrium

Many delicate sensory systems function together to maintain equilibrium. These include the vestibules, retina, and proprioceptive receptors in the neck muscles, muscles and ligaments of the foot, and many other sites throughout the body, even the abdominal omentum.

Information from all these sensory systems and receptors is collected at the level of the vestibular nuclei, which are responsible for vestibular-ocular reflexes, for example, adaptive shifting of the eye in order to maintain lateral vision. When these reflexes are disrupted, nystagmus results.

The spinal cord sends impulses to the vestibular nuclei, triggering vestibular-spinal reflexes. Harmonization of postural muscular adjustments is essential for maintenance of balance and execution of movements.

Movement sensations originate from the thalamus and the frontal and occipital cortex.

The cerebellum controls the vestibular-ocular and vestibular-spinal reflex pathways via the Purkinje cells of the flocculus. The flocculus is essential for maintaining an image on the retina; if it is damaged, the image becomes disjointed.

Symptoms of disturbances of pathways governing equilibrium

- true vertigo with a sense of directional imbalance triggered by movements of the head and neck. Very rarely, there is severe rotatory paroxysmal vertigo. This differs from Ménière's vertigo because of the absence of deafness.
- ocular or visual problems like hemianopsia (scotoma in less than half the visual field of one or both eyes), cortical blindness, photopsia
- paresthesia of the upper or lower extremities, face, tongue, or mouth
- headaches, posterior at first, then radiating to the orbits
- problems with awareness, memory, or language
- dysarthria
- vestibulocochlear syndrome

Posterior inferior cerebellar artery syndrome

This is a transient ischemic attack of the cerebral artery due to thrombosis of the vertebral artery, also known as Wallenberg's syndrome. Characteristic signs include:

- severe rotatory vertigo with vomiting, headaches, or hiccups
- problems with speech and swallowing
- a staggering gait, and sensation of being "pushed" toward the side of the lesion

- vertical or oblique diplopia caused by a difference in level of the two eyes (ipsilateral eye is lower)
- ipsilateral facial hemianesthesia
- velar-pharyngeal hemiplegia
- ipsilateral Horner's syndrome, with contralateral loss of sensitivity to pain and temperature.

Premenstrual and perimenopausal vertigo

Premenstrual vertigo typically does not appear until around 40 years of age. It is probably caused by faulty calcium metabolism in the inner ear, edema of the inner ear, or Ménière's disease.

We see many premenopausal or menopausal women who suffer from vertigo, usually caused by decompensation of hormonal origin. Liver function is often disturbed during menopause, due to poor elimination of estrogens, which increases the likelihood of vertigo.

We had a patient who, at age 25, suffered craniocervical trauma during a fall from a hay wagon. Every four or five years she came to us with a complaint of headaches, but it was not until age 47 that intense vertigo appeared.

Various practitioners attributed psychological causes to this vertigo, including her unwillingness to grow old and her desire to "remain a woman." However, the numerous treatments that they prescribed were useless. We made her vertigo disappear entirely by releasing the attachments of the ligaments of the right clavicle and T2. This case showed an interesting association among trauma, menopause, and muscular/ligamentous restrictions.

Vertigo from motion sickness

Motion sickness is a "sensory conflict" resulting when the vestibular, visual, and proprioceptive sensors stimulated by the body's movements send discordant information to the integrative vestibular nuclei.

In motion sickness, the vestibular nuclei seem to receive excessive stimuli from the eyes, neck, and cerebellum. People suffering from motion sickness often have hypersensitive gallbladders, or various problems with liver function.

Poor bile metabolism is one of numerous factors—including trauma, infection, anxiety, liver and gallbladder problems, age, hormone imbalance, and travel—which in combination can produce vertigo.

Vertigo from epileptic seizures

We are speaking not about grand mal seizures, which have been well-studied and documented, but rather small epileptiform seizures undetectable by EEG, CAT scan, or MRI. We see these often in our practice, after cranial or, less often, cervical trauma.

These seizures may result from electrical malfunction of the CNS, or tiny cranial scars capable of creating electrical discharges. These phenomena increase in association with exertion, anger, pain, large changes in temperature, stormy weather, and the like.

We had a patient who, following a painful ankle sprain, complained of vertigo and headaches. Ten years earlier he had a craniocervical trauma without any apparent effects. His sprain had caused a decompensation of his adaptation to his previous trauma, leading to the symptoms which brought him to our office.

Transient Ischemic Attacks (TIAs)

This is a focal neurological deficit, secondary to a cerebral ischemia, which clears in less than 24 hours. TIAs can result from certain craniocervical traumas, but there are many other possible causes to be considered.

Pathogenesis

TIAs are usually caused by embolism following atheromatous lesions in the arteries above the level of the aorta. An embolus breaks loose from a platelet mass or thrombus, which is often friable. The embolus causes transient ischemia by reducing the arterial diameter and blood flow.

Causes

Atheromatous emboli are the most common type of embolus, found in patients with a vascular atheromatous predisposition.

Cardiac problems responsible for TIAs are cardiopathy, valvular disease, dysrhythmia, or endocarditis.

Other causes include arterial dissection, hypertension, diabetes, tobacco use (especially associated with oral contraceptives), high cholesterol, and obesity.

Signs

TIAs are sudden, usually established in less than a minute, and regress spontaneously within five minutes. Signs and symptoms depend on the areas affected.

Basilar area

- sensory/motor problems of one or more extremities and the face
- visual field problems
- ataxia and balance problems without vertigo
- drop attacks (collapse of lower extremities while fully conscious)

Carotid area

- transient monocular blindness, due to ischemia of the ophthalmic artery
- motor problems producing hemiparesis, sometimes only at the level of the hand or torso
- unilateral sensory problems (paresthesia, hypoesthesia, astereognosis)
- problems with language, including inability to express oneself or to understand others

TIAs in young people

We see such cases only when symptoms are slight. The main causes are tearing of cervical arteries, cardiac abnormalities, oral contraceptives, tobacco use, migraines, infections, and trauma (a triggering factor). The ratio of cerebral infarcts to TIAs in young people is roughly two to one. Causes of TIAs include the following.

Arterial tears

These affect the carotid and vertebral arteries, and are either spontaneous or due to trauma. There is no arterial hypertension.

Cardiac abnormalities

Frequent causes of cardiopathy are emboli, valve implants, mitral stenosis, and mitral valve prolapse. Less frequent causes are patent foramen ovale and cardiomegaly.

Other causes of TIAs

Tobacco use, oral contraceptives, arterial hypertension, diabetes, high cholesterol, migraine, presence of antiphospholipid antibodies, infections (e.g., meningitis, endocarditis), or trauma (a triggering factor).

Conclusion

We have covered a large variety of illnesses, syndromes, and symptoms in this chapter because you will sometimes encounter complex cases which require immediate referral to a specialist. Here is one example.

Mr. X, 41 years old, a hard-working professional, suffered a slight cervical sprain as he arrived at work. He came to us for cervical pain associated with a sense of instability, slight loss of equilibrium, and severe anxiety.

Physical examination did not reveal any major osseous, muscular, or ligamentous restrictions. There was a large sternal scar from an operation for mitral stenosis which occurred at age 14.

Given the lack of vertebral restrictions, the symptoms of instability and severe anxiety, and the cardiac surgical history, we referred Mr. X to a cardiologist who diagnosed a small embolus at the level of the basilar artery. In such cases we must be alert for certain diseases or symptoms in order to establish a differential diagnosis. It is important to know our limitations as osteopaths, and to realize when a specialist is needed.

Psychic and Emotional Reactions to Trauma

In order to distinguish between psychic reactions and emotional ones, we need to define *psyche* and *emotion*.

- The psyche is all the structures and content of the conscious and unconscious mind which combine to create the "self."
- Emotion is a mental reaction or disturbance elicited by a pleasant or unpleasant event, often accompanied by physical manifestations.

A psychic reaction to trauma affects the deepest part of the victim's person, while an emotional reaction is merely a manifestation in response to a problem. In serious cases, the emotions and the psyche interact.

Emotional reactions

Characteristics

THEY CAN BE SPONTANEOUS OR DELAYED

Immediately after the accident, emotional reactions can include crying, dejection, "lump in the throat," collapse, hyperexcitability, rage, desire for revenge, and loss of self-control.

THEY ARE STORED IN MEMORY

Emotional reactions may develop over the course of days, weeks, or even months following the trauma. Some subjects appear not to be marked by the trauma experienced. Whether they are expressed or not, however, emotional reactions are stored in memory and become part of the subject's emotional history.

Memory storage of trauma is at the level of the cerebral centers, and perhaps also in the tissues which have suffered. The latter phenomenon is referred to as tissue memory. We cannot definitively prove it, but various clinical observations would appear to confirm its existence.

THEY ARE CUMULATIVE AND FACILITATED

When the limbic or paralimbic centers are stimulated, they trigger emotional reactions. These new stimuli in turn awaken other emotional memories stored in the brain. This explains cases of disproportionate reaction to a minor trauma. The emotion of the slight trauma has been added to the previous emotions.

Take the example of a man who witnesses a serious automobile accident in which one of the victims bleeds profusely. Suppose that later this man cuts his finger slightly. The mere vision of the few drops of blood is capable of triggering a syncope or other serious reaction because of the cumulative and facilitative properties of the emotions.

An emotion which is experienced on top of other stored emotions may create unexpected reactions. We call these "facilitated emotional reactions" in analogy to physiological facilitated segments. A good example is a patient of ours who unexpectedly saw a snake in front of her. In the process of jumping back to avoid it, she fell on her coccyx. The sacral/coccygeal trauma thus became associated with a fear of snakes. Several years later, the patient knocked her sacral region lightly against a table while rearranging her house. She began to cry uncontrollably and subsequently fell into a depression. Several phenomena combined to produce this effect:

- the physical pain
- the memory in the sacral/coccygeal tissues
- the central emotional memory
- her entire psycho-emotional history.

THEY ARE PURELY REACTIVE

Emotions follow and result from some event. They are rarely spontaneous, in contrast to psychic reactions. They need a physical or psychic triggering factor in order to reappear.

Localization

TISSUE EMOTIONAL MEMORY

Simply touching an injured area can trigger a serious emotional reaction. Some might say that the area touched merely acts as a trigger by sending proprioceptive stimuli to the central nerves. However, we believe that the tissue itself can serve as an "emotional warehouse."

This is quite difficult to prove scientifically. How can one follow neural input of this nature? PET scans may some day allow better understanding of this phenomenon.

They can show the activity of certain limbic areas, but not of the body tissues themselves. Some say that what we call "tissue memory" is a result of stimulation of the central emotional areas; however, tissues are far from having revealed all their secrets. Just think of the "unused" information capacity of DNA and RNA.

Central emotional memory

At the level of the CNS, emotional or general memory appears to be localized in several areas of the brain. Of these, the limbic system and hippocampus are the best documented.

In our manual approach to emotional disturbances, we have located one major cerebral center deep in the anteromedial portion of the right parietal lobe, next to the sagittal suture and behind the coronal suture (see *Manual Thermal Diagnosis*, page 65). This corresponds roughly to the topography of the limbic system.

Psychic reactions

Although it is often impossible to separate emotional reactions from psychic ones, general distinctions do exist. Emotional reactions are direct, not very well elaborated, and more easily compensated. Psychic reactions are more complex and are pathogenic.

Characteristics of a psychic reaction

It affects the inner being

A psychic reaction is not proportional to the severity of the trauma. The external features of a trauma (severity of lesions, spectacular aspect of the accident, reactions of surrounding people) have a minimal effect on the "inner being," compared to the effect of the victim's own reactions.

It is a rejection of reality

Lacan (1972) noted that at the time of an accident, reality appears in a form that is impossible to take in. Thus, the victim can neither accept nor compensate for the event. It is a "failed meeting with death."

It is an encounter with mortality

Death, and the fear of death, are inherent parts of our lives. Any trauma conveys an image of our mortality, which we repel or reject. In the words of Woody Allen, "As long as he is mortal, man can never be really relaxed." An accident forces us to confront the idea of death. The victim of an accident will "relive" it over and over, sometimes adding details or otherwise embellishing her memories of it. These embellishments can include other things that the subject is afraid of, even though they were not actually part of the particular trauma.

It creates a rupture of psychosomatic integrity

In order to function effectively, an individual requires "psychosomatic integrity." He lives as if in a sort of enclosure, which belongs to him and must remain inviolate. This enclosure is an indispensable protection for the relationship between the body and psyche. When trauma occurs, the enclosure is broken and the harmonious relationship disrupted. The effects of this are more severe when there is an outsider involved.

It devalues us

In the simple example of an assault by another person, the break in the enclosure is more complex. In addition to the harmful effects described above, there is an additional feeling of being devalued by the other party and by oneself. In many cases, the subsequent self-devaluation arises from having suffered the assault passively. The French saying *On est peu de choses* ("how insignificant a thing man is") conveys this feeling.

It lays the blame on us

During trauma, the instinct for self-preservation makes us react spontaneously and instinctively in order to protect ourselves. Later, our various ties to others, and society, remind us of our moral and financial responsibilities. This is when we begin to blame ourselves. This is a thought-out reaction, and can have serious repercussions.

It is indelible

Post-traumatic psychic reactions are more hierarchic, elaborate, and intense than emotional reactions, and create an indelible trace in the psychic centers. This trace is more serious and more pathogenic than that from an emotional reaction. A patient who confronts and fears death has been marked for life, her subconscious mind imprinted. Even if treatment is successful and the patient feels and functions better, she is still marked by the experience.

It can reappear spontaneously

Old emotional reactions usually reappear following a more recent emotion. In the case of psychic reactions, they often resurface suddenly and spontaneously, for no apparent reason.

Psycho-emotional interdependence

When trauma is severe, emotional and psychic reactions intermingle, producing an indelible mark on the conscious, and more importantly, on the subconscious, mind of the victim.

The subconscious seems capable of recording events which occur in a thousandth of a second! The stories told to us by patients are amazing. Some have been able to recount in great detail the unfolding of the accident, as well as noises, odors, behaviors of other people—partly during a period when the patient was unconscious.

As osteopaths, we can free up certain emotions which have become buried in order to help rid the patient of psycho-emotional shackles. Freedom from these emotions allows the psyche to function better. We have the ability to lighten the psychic and emotional "load." When the reactions are more psychic than emotional, it is better to refer the patient to a psychologist or psychiatrist. Most of us do not possess sufficient competence in this area to be sure that we are, if fact, doing no harm.

Chapter Five:
Diagnosis

Table of Contents

Diagnosis

General Remarks

Osteopathic diagnosis is a difficult process to summarize because there are so many types and causes of restrictions. As explained in our previous books, a good osteopathic diagnosis requires knowing how to "listen" to the body and allow the hand to be drawn to the affected tissues. Listening enables us to locate and analyze tissue tensions or restrictions, although this task is not as easy as it may sound!

As osteopaths, we do not give priority to symptoms described by the patient, but do take them into account to guide our interpretation of manual listening. "The tree which falls makes more noise than the entire growing forest," according to the ancient Chinese proverb. A complaint of lower back pain may be merely the tree hiding the forest, for example, rupture of an ovarian cyst.

Some important properties (and sources of difficulty!) in osteopathic diagnosis are discussed below.

"Nothing is forgotten"

All stresses, whether physical or psychoemotional, are retained in the body's memory. A fall on the coccyx in early childhood can leave a long trace in certain tissues. The fall is part of the subject's history and will likely have future pathological consequences.

"Nothing is isolated"

A trauma to any part of the body can affect any other part. The fall on the coccyx causes a shock wave capable of spreading to any tissue. If you have experienced this, you may remember an impression of a moving cerebral mass when the shock wave reached the skull, or a feeling of intense heat or combustion in certain parts of the body.

"Everything accumulates"

Any stress to the body is recorded in the tissues, remembered, and sometimes even amplified. A healthy body has numerous mechanisms for adaptation and compensation, and trauma may not cause obvious lesions or symptoms. On the other hand, if the body has exhausted its possibilities for compensation, even a slight stress is capable of triggering severe symptoms.

We have seen severe cervicobrachial neuralgia with paresthesia and signs of neurological deficits as a result of a simple blow to the skull. Cervical x-rays demonstrated foraminal shrinking of the vertebral segment in question, but the condition had existed for years without noticeable symptoms. This phenomenon is well known in our field; it is analogous to that one drop of water that causes a vase to overflow.

"Everything is recorded"

Prelesional zones

These are zones of asymptomatic lesions which may develop anywhere in the body. For example, arthrosis does not arise spontaneously, but develops in joints that have been mechanically stressed or injured. Irvin Korr's (1978) concept of facilitated segments in the spinal cord is similar. For example, an irritated stomach bombards its corresponding spinal segment (T6-T7) with nervous stimuli. This segment is facilitated and will react to even a small stimulus from a distant part of the body. In this way, a trauma to the knee can cause thoracic restrictions.

Another example is the patient who develops acute sciatica after simple coughing or sneezing. In this case, the shock wave from the cough or sneeze is concentrated on a prelesional zone at the corresponding discoforaminal junction.

Zones of fetal predisposition

Many of our patients are pregnant women, and we have had the opportunity to test the position of the fetus *in utero* to determine possible zones of compression or decreased mobility, and to check our findings by testing the child's skull after birth. We have always found restrictions in the newborn where the skull was constrained *in utero*.

Cranial or spinal restrictions resulting from fetal malpositioning cause a morbid "lateral tendency" in which the subject repeatedly hurts himself on the side where the fetal stress occurred. There may also be a genetic predisposition to this tendency. Genetics is a field which is beginning to explain formerly inexplicable phenomena. Is illness predetermined? Is everything prerecorded? We cannot answer such fundamental questions at this time, yet we do not believe that lesions occur completely at random!

Importance and nature of the lesion

The importance of a lesion should not be judged based on "quantity." Sometimes a slight fall or movement is capable of destabilizing the body and causing significant pain, while a seemingly severe trauma can pass almost unnoticed. As an example, a logger was hit on the head by a tree trunk. The force of the impact literally shattered the entire right squamoparietal area. The neurosurgeon who operated was content to remove the osseous fragments and suture the dura mater to cover and protect the brain. This patient did not subsequently suffer from headaches, dizziness, or fatigue. Each time he came for a consultation we were able to feel cranial movement *only in contact with the bone!* Direct manual contact with the dura mater revealed nothing.

"Body and mind"

Somatization

There is a delicate balance between the psychoemotional and physical systems. When patients describe symptoms that are not objectively demonstrable, some practitioners attribute the symptoms to somatization, that is, projecting a psychological disturbance onto the body.

Such patients are often told that the pain is "all in their mind," or are treated with condescension by the medical establishment. However, we obviously cannot feel our patients' pain for them. When pain appears, it is neither objective, nor subjective, nor real, nor imagined; it simply "is."

A certain degree of somatization is desirable, as it reflects body-mind communication. A healthy individual finds the proper balance between her body and mind. Anything that affects one will affect the other. Osteopathy, a global type of medicine, treats body and mind together.

Osteopathic "lesions" and "restrictions"

The lesion which we treat is part of a whole and difficult to isolate. We prefer the older term "osteopathic lesion" over the newer term used in American osteopathic medicine, "somatic dysfunction," which we feel is more limited. The osteopathic concept of restriction is a global concept of disruption in the proper motion of tissues, which may stem from multiple causes. The tissues lose their mobility, motility, and energy.

To differentiate them from the tissue lesions of conventional medicine, we use the term "restriction" when discussing these reductions in motion. Restrictions are found by osteopaths using their hands. They are often unrecognized by conventional medicine, or are called by different names. Unfortunately, the dichotomy in labeling can adversely affect communication between osteopaths and conventional medical practitioners.

State of good health

We can illustrate our concept of good health by a scale with two sides, each capable of being tilted in the direction of either poor or good health *(Fig. 5-1)*. At the left are listed negative factors which may occur during the life of the individual. No one is impervious to restrictions, yet as long as the forces of compensation and adaptation are operative, the negative factors are well compensated for, and the subject is in good health. More precisely, she is in *a state of apparent good health*, in other words, without any symptoms.

Trauma may be represented by a weight. Depending on the position of the balance scale just beforehand, a small traumatic weight may be sufficient to upset the equilibrium of balance and move the patient into illness. That is, if the forces of compensation or adaptation are near their limit, even a slight negative event can trigger illness. Once again we can use the analogy of the last drop of water which causes the vase to overflow. This phenomenon explains how a mild cold can develop into pneumonia, or picking a pin off the floor can cause acute lower back pain, or a simple lack of success in love can lead to severe depression.

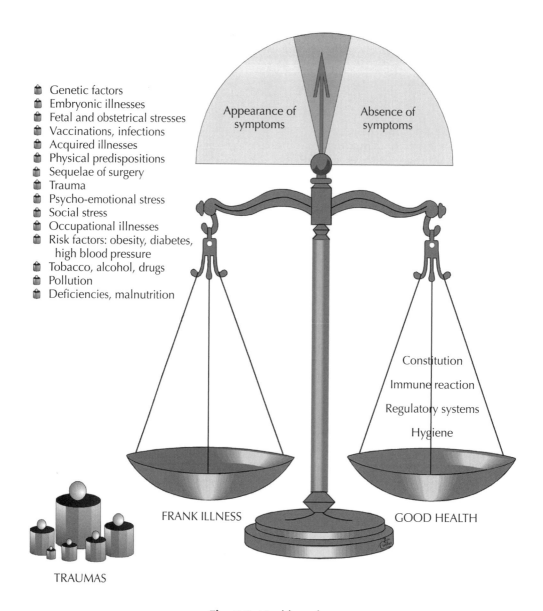

- Genetic factors
- Embryonic illnesses
- Fetal and obstetrical stresses
- Vaccinations, infections
- Acquired illnesses
- Physical predispositions
- Sequelae of surgery
- Trauma
- Psycho-emotional stress
- Social stress
- Occupational illnesses
- Risk factors: obesity, diabetes, high blood pressure
- Tobacco, alcohol, drugs
- Pollution
- Deficiencies, malnutrition

Appearance of symptoms

Absence of symptoms

Constitution

Immune reaction

Regulatory systems

Hygiene

FRANK ILLNESS

GOOD HEALTH

TRAUMAS

Fig. 5-1: Health scales

The lesions which may be improved by osteopathic care are numerous and varied. They include fetal stress and its consequences, sequelae of abnormal childbirth, trauma, and certain psychoactive stresses which can be released by the body with the help of manipulation.

Fig. 5-1 also mentions social stress, of which unemployment is a perfect example. An individual who still has adaptation and compensation reserves can react positively to the loss of a job. On the other hand, if he has reached his adaptation/compensation limit, he may develop such problems as an ulcer, depression, acute lower back pain, or infection.

Many other negative factors affecting the "health scale" remain unknown. Medical progress was greatly advanced by the discovery of bacteria, viruses, and prions. What secrets will be unlocked by the next major medical discovery?

Note: We include vaccinations in the list of negative factors not because we oppose them, but because some of them can prove problematic in a predisposing environment. The DTP vaccine, for example, sharply decreases craniosacral motion in certain children for a long period of time. These children become easily fatigued, experience significant learning problems, and may develop a variety of mild respiratory or allergic illnesses.

The General Examination

Each osteopath has a personal approach to the general exam. We do not intend to give strict rules or describe all possible procedures. We will simply focus on some important points relevant to osteopathic diagnosis and treatment of trauma.

The interview

Aside from the immediate reason for consultation, one goal of the osteopathic interview is to uncover all the traumatic incidents which may have affected the patient during his life. Manual diagnosis reveals to us the extent to which each incident has left its imprint on the patient's tissues. We must determine if the consequences of the trauma account for the symptomatology, and if they are within our competence to treat.

It is of course important to find out the circumstances of the accident, evaluation performed, appearance of pain, type of pain, periodicity, and so forth. However, it is equally important to be aware that *the trauma may be the tree which hides the forest.* Trauma can awaken other well-compensated traumatic tissue sequelae and can, importantly, reveal a latent asymptomatic illness on the point of manifesting itself. This is why it is important to discover any clinical signs or symptoms the patient had before the accident.

Interpretation of the word "trauma" varies widely among people. We must adapt our vocabulary according to the case at hand and use synonyms such as blow, impact, fall, accident, and so on. We personally like to ask the patient to describe any "memorable" falls, impacts, or blows.

Except in cases of traffic accidents, sports, falls, or "significant" impacts, patients usually have no memory of the initial trauma, or do not associate it with long-term symptoms or distant repercussions. For this reason, you should always cover traumatic antecedents during the interview. You can jog the patient's memory by mentioning possible etiologies, for example:

- sports (especially contact sports and martial arts)
- traffic accidents (automobile, bicycle, motorcycle, pedestrian)
- workplace accidents
- leisure accidents (gardening, hunting, fishing, touring)
- falls from a height.

If possible, try to find out the location of the impact or whiplash, and the position of the body and head at the time.

Significant problems ("delayed trauma") may occur long after the initial event. Visceral rupture may occur in two phases; for example, a kidney or spleen may rupture 40 days after the original injury!

Investigation of traumatic antecedents should always be included in the interview, regardless of the reason for consultation. It never ceases to amaze us that a person's entire life can be altered by a traumatic event that occurs in one brief instant.

Blood pressure and pulse

Asymmetric pressure

Always check the blood pressure of trauma patients. An unusual drop in pressure may signify a micro-hemorrhage which was missed during previous examinations, a CNS dysfunction, or the beginning of post-traumatic depression.

Asymmetric pressure often results from visceral, osteoarticular, or tissue problems. The phenomenon permits objective assessment if blood pressure is measured before and after treatment. If our treatment was effective, the pressures on the right and left sides become more symmetric.

The pulse

A rapid, indistinct pulse accompanied by significant pallor, nausea, and fainting indicates a problem requiring careful and precise diagnosis, and perhaps referral for emergency care. We have noted small hemorrhages in cases of post-traumatic skull edema, or after fractures, which evaded diagnosis by other practitioners.

A difference between the two pulses often indicates an osteoarticular problem affecting the balance between the parasympathetic and sympathetic nervous systems. The problem is usually located on the side where the pulse is least noticeable. Another common reason for this type of phenomenon is a decrease in the functional lumen of the subclavian or axillary arteries. This compression can be due to an anatomical compression or a change in the sympathetic tone affecting them.

Exaggerated abdominal aortic pulse

This usually signifies intense anxiety, but very rarely may be a sign of a spontaneous or post-traumatic aortic aneurysm. When this is the case, the pulse is easily felt (and sometimes seen) throughout the abdominal cavity. One of the first signs of an aortic aneurysm is a low-grade thoracic or lumbar pain that arises spontaneously without any mechanical cause-and-effect relationship.

Adson-Wright test

This test, used frequently in osteopathy, enables us to locate the zone of restriction and evaluate its development. The patient is in a seated position, with arms hanging down and shoulders relaxed. Standing behind the patient, with one knee on the table, take the patient's wrists to draw the forearm and arms into "candlestick position" (abduction and external rotation of the glenohumeral joint).

During the manipulation, your index and middle fingers evaluate the quality of the radial pulse, which should remain constant. Any variation in or disappearance of the pulse indicates an ipsilateral restriction. Except in true thoracic inlet restrictions with compression of the subclavian artery between the clavicle and first rib, variation in the radial pulse is a reflex vasoconstrictive phenomenon. In the case of cervical whiplash, simply compressing the cervical spine by pressing the top of the skull may cause the radial pulse to vary during this test.

Palpation

In addition to osteopathic tissue palpation, be on the lookout for nodes, cervical or subclavicular cutaneous emphysema, abnormally strong pulsation of the abdominal aorta, or sharp visceral or tissue pain. These are all signs of conditions which require prompt evaluation by conventional means.

Lymph nodes

Enlarged lymph nodes may be cervical, subclavicular, axillary, or inguinal. They usually reflect immune system reaction to an infection or tumor, but can also be a sign of extreme generalized fatigue.

PALPATION OF NODES AND SWELLINGS OF THE NECK

While palpating the cervical spine, neck, and subclavian fossae during examinations, we commonly encounter small areas of enlarged nodes. These are usually benign, but occasionally prove to be malignant. If you have any doubt about this, refer the patient for evaluation. Cervical pain of mechanical origin *per se* very rarely causes nodes, although nodes are often accompanied by cervical pain which reveals other underlying pathological conditions.

In many cases, the consequences of trauma are accompanied by infection or other pathologies which the trauma helps unmask. An example is an asymptomatic cervical metastasis in a patient suffering from whiplash. The cervical pain seems to be a normal reaction to the trauma and may mask the tumor process. However, because there are nodes, you will request imaging studies before initiating any treatment, and these will reveal the tumor.

NODE LOCATION AND ADENOPATHY

Each node location reflects problems in different parts of the body:

- submandibular and submental nodes: problems of the anterior tongue, gums and buccal areas, or zygomatic areas
- subparotid and lateral superficial cervical nodes: problems of the tonsils, base of tongue, salivary glands, teeth, gums, nose, eyes, and ears
- anterior cervical nodes: pathology of the tongue, tonsils, nasopharynx, larynx, middle ear, parotid, thyroid, and (less frequently) the mediastinal/esophageal region
- posterior cervical nodes: abrasions and infections of the lower scalp or nape of the neck, dental problems, colds, and influenzas. Also common in children approaching adolescence. May indicate depressed immune resistance from prolonged fatigue or other causes. We also observe them in women with postpartum iron deficiency or excessive menstrual flow.

Note: For inflammatory cervical pain with nodes and low-grade fever, but without significant vertebral restriction, manipulation is *contraindicated.*

Not all swellings in the jaw or neck area are lymph nodes. The parotid glands are felt as a swelling in the subauricular retromaxillary groove, or behind the ramus of the mandible. The thyroid can cause lower cervical pain, especially in the case of hyper-thyroidism and goiter, and should be palpated during the exam.

ACUTE ADENOPATHY

If the nodes are sensitive and painful to palpation, this may indicate infectious disease, for example, localized ulcerations or dental, buccolingual, or pharyngeal infections.

NONACUTE ADENOPATHY

With *mononucleosis*, nodes are only slightly sensitive or completely painless. They are felt at the cervical level, in the axillary fossa, and inguinal grooves.

With *measles*, nodes are retroauricular, cervical, and occipital.

Chauffard's syndrome is a chronic, evolving polyarthritis of childhood. It is characterized by high fever and signs of systemic illness which may exist for months before the onset of any joint pain. The nodes are hypertrophied, firm, and mobile, and can be palpated at the cervical, axillary, and inguinal levels.

PSEUDO-INFECTIOUS ADENOPATHY

With *Hodgkin's disease*, we find unilateral anteroinferior cervical nodes, which later become bilateral and spread to other lymph node regions. The nodes are resilient, regular, mobile, and painless. Eventually, splenomegaly develops, with severe adenopathy, itching, fluctuating temperature, and other characteristic signs.

Acute leukemias cause cervical polyadenitis.

Lymphosarcoma begins with a single firm node. Subsequent adenopathy of the surrounding area sometimes forms a large, irregular mass which may be either soft or hard.

Asymptomatic adenopathies give rise to small, resilient, elastic nodes which are non-adherent, mobile, and painless. They may result from asymptomatic dental problems or infections, or from chronic fatigue. "Subclinical" infectious states sometimes occur when growth exhausts the adolescent patient and depresses the immunological defenses.

ISOLATED ANTERIOR CERVICAL MASS

These are malignant in 50% of cases! They occur most frequently in smokers and drinkers around 55-years of age. The masses are usually larger than 2cm and located at the anterior cervical or subclavicular region. They are hard, irritating, or painful, and increase rapidly in size. In cases of esophageal cancer, swallowing and voice are affected.

GENERALIZATIONS ABOUT LYMPH NODES

These may be helpful in your practice, but be aware that there are always exceptions!

- A mass under the chin is usually benign.
- A cervical mass of 2cm or more is often malignant.
- A subclavicular mass should be considered malignant until proven otherwise.

Palpation of the cervical and clavicular regions can be confusing. Many structures are easy to mistake for nodes:

- C1 transverse process
- C2 spinous process
- large transverse process of a lower cervical vertebra
- short cervical rib
- greater horn of hyoid bone
- atheromatous carotid sinus
- subclavicular lipoma (more frequent in women and on the left side)
- a large dolichoectatic artery off the brachiocephalic trunk (pulsatile mass located in the right subclavicular groove).

Cutaneous emphysema

A crackling sensation of the soft tissues of the neck or subclavicular region upon palpation may indicate pneumothorax. Get a chest x-ray immediately. Do not attempt to manipulate the first or lower ribs!

Objective examinations

The guiding principle in osteopathic treatment is "First, do no harm." Extreme care must be taken with trauma patients. The statement "The worst x-rays are sometimes worth more than the best pair of hands" applies to these patients.

Never begin treatment of a trauma patient until she has had the appropriate objective examinations. Keep in mind that some examinations, performed hastily in overcrowded emergency rooms, may not be reliable.

In this section we will discuss aspects of imaging technologies relevant to our own clinical practice, and treatment of trauma patients.

X-ray

X-rays are most useful for evaluating the integrity of bony structures. However, the accuracy of this objective procedure is greatly dependent on the competence of the technician. A major limitation is that x-ray does not reveal soft tissues, that is, arteries, veins, lymph vessels, muscles, ligaments, cartilage, or nerves. Only extravasion of blood in soft tissues may be visible, due to the increased density it creates. If x-rays are "negative," this usually signifies only that the bones are in good shape.

There are many potential sources of error in diagnosis based on x-ray.

- The technician uses specific orientations of the instrument or body part in search of lesions, but neglects others.
- Preexisting conditions are mistaken for effects of trauma without prior x-ray records for comparison.
- Undetectability of an osseous lesion.
- The period of time that elapses between the trauma and the x-ray. Certain fractures, for example, of ribs and wrist bones, are visible only after several days, because of bony reabsorption at the focal site.

- Quality of the x-ray film or equipment. Some clinics, or parts of the world, have better technology than others. Be very careful when treating victims of an accident which occurred in an underdeveloped country!
- Technician error resulting in poor quality images.
- The injured area is not investigated. We have seen cases of humeral fractures which were not diagnosed initially, because only the spine was subjected to x-ray. We are influenced by what the patient tells us. Intense pain in one area may mask injury in a different, less painful area.

Try to obtain an interpretative summary by a qualified radiologist. A hurriedly given oral report is obviously not as reliable as a written summary, which requires a very different mind set.

Routine, standard x-rays may be insufficient. If you have doubt, send the patient for more sophisticated imaging studies. Specialized procedures such as tomography, dynamic imaging, or scintigraphy may be the only way to reveal the true diagnosis following trauma.

We treat many spinal trauma patients. Spinal cord injury has many possible causes, including concussion, contusion, compression, tear, or extravasion of blood. Be on the lookout for signs of these on x-ray.

CT, MRI, and PET scans

These can be useful examinations for imaging the viscera or nervous system and establishing a diagnosis when x-rays are negative or difficult to interpret.

The computerized tomography (CT) scan (sometimes with addition of contrast media) permits imaging of swelling of the cerebral ventricles, in addition to dense structures. It should be done as soon as possible for victims of cerebral trauma in order to establish the need for rapid surgical intervention. It is the tool of choice for diagnosis of intracranial hematoma, a serious complication of cranial trauma, and permits us to distinguish hemorrhage from cerebral ischemic attacks.

Magnetic resonance imaging (MRI) is a precise structural technique for examination of the brain and brainstem, often used in cases of traumatic coma. It permits us to follow changes of cerebral tissue over time, and to refine diagnosis or prognosis.

Positron emission tomography (PET) permits determination of different rates of metabolism of different areas of the brain, and evaluation of cerebral metabolism of patients with prolonged coma.

These techniques are used only when absolutely necessary, and available. The machines, and experienced people to run them, are limited and expensive, even in developed countries. Results must be evaluated by specialists.

Ultrasound

In cases of abdominal trauma, this minimally invasive procedure is often the method of choice to evaluate visceral integrity. Ultrasound is the best objective technique to reveal rupture of the spleen, which is common following trauma, and is often useful to diagnose an internal hemorrhage. Ultrasound is one of the few methods for diagnosing muscular and tendinous lesions, including extravasion inside tissue, tendinous rupture, and intramuscular hematoma.

A visceral rupture often occurs in two phases following trauma to the abdomen, thorax, or lumbar wall. The first phase is a small injury accompanied by little bleeding.

After some time (possibly several days), pressure inside the organ increases from the bleeding and there is a secondary rupture which gives rise to internal hemorrhage.

Organ rupture can occur without serious trauma. An injury as slight as banging against a table after a meal can cause rupture of the stomach. The subject experiences severe and persistent epigastric pain, and vomiting. X-ray of the abdomen reveals pneumoperitonitis, and ultrasound confirms extravasation.

Ultrasound is also the method of choice for diagnosing trauma of the pancreas. The most common causes are car accidents in adults, and bicycle accidents in children. Minor trauma or blows may also be responsible. The body of the pancreas is injured at the point where it crosses the spine. The lesion may consist of a simple contusion, formation of a hemorrhagic pseudocyst, or a prevertebral rupture of the organ. Rupture may occur in two phases as described above, with a delay of several days or even months before the second phase. These examples demonstrate the importance of avoiding delay when dealing with visceral ruptures.

The Osteopathic Examination

Introduction

Detection of traumatic lesions

Osteopathy and conventional medicine differ greatly in their approach to trauma. Conventional medical diagnosis relies upon objective inspection and analysis. For a long time, articular medical diagnosis relied upon radiography. In other words, diagnosis was based solely upon what was visible upon x-ray and completely immobile.

Aside from fractures and significant fluid extravasation, which are visible on x-ray, all abnormalities involving the muscles, tendons, connective tissue, joint capsules, synovial membranes, arteries, veins, and nerves are missed by this type of diagnosis. Ultrasound and MRI permit us to view some soft tissues, but do not yield information on changes in mobility, tone, motility, or functioning.

Primary role of the hand

A basic principle of osteopathy is that practitioners not only see but also feel with their hands. Palpation, motion testing, and manual listening are essential parts of our diagnostic approach. The patient interview is important, yet we cannot always expect the patient to tell us the location of her major problem. Relying solely on symptomatology often leads to misdiagnosis. The hand is most capable of diagnosing tissue injuries of the body. Manual diagnosis lets the body "speak" and give its own information about mobility.

In Europe, osteopathy is an office-based practice, and we typically see sequelae of trauma. Osteopaths do not work in emergency care centers. Fractures, parenchymatous degeneration and the like are initially diagnosed and treated in a hospital or the clinic of a conventional physician.

Objective evidence confirming manual diagnosis

A frequent problem in communicating with conventional medical practitioners is that it is difficult to objectively document most of our findings. We occasionally manage to confirm our diagnosis through conventional means, for example, with renal ptoses, changes in CSF pressure, small pneumothorax, undetected fractures, and minor cerebral lesions. However, these are isolated cases. There is no technology yet that can confirm most of what is felt by trained hands. It is significant that osteopaths from different countries with different types of training will usually reach the same diagnosis for a given patient. This has been our experience in Europe, Australia, the United States, Japan, and Russia.

Dura mater diagnosis

The spinal cord is suspended in the fibrous dura mater sac. After opening the spinal canal during a dissection, it is easy to separate the dura mater from the spinal cord to display the posterior surface of the vertebral body *(Fig. 5-2)*. Aside from the dentate ligaments by which it is joined to the other meningeal layers, the spinal dura mater is linked:

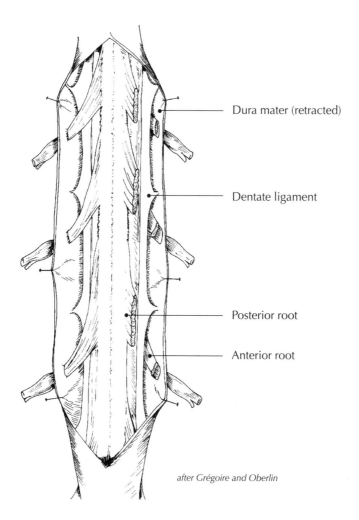

Dura mater (retracted)

Dentate ligament

Posterior root

Anterior root

after Grégoire and Oberlin

Fig. 5-2: The dura mater and spinal roots

- *anteriorly*, to the posterior common vertebral ligament by several fibrous projections
- *laterally*, to the intervertebral foramen, by the sheaths surrounding the spinal nerves, or the perineurium *(Fig. 5-3)*
- *posteriorly*, to the parietal layer of the arachnoid
- *at its superior end*, to the posterior surface of the body of the axis, and the periphery of the foramen magnum where it joins the cranial dura mater
- *at its inferior end*, to the sacrum (S2-S3), terminating in the deep posterior sacrococcygeal ligament, an extension of the posterior longitudinal ligament at the coccygeal level *(Fig. 5-4)*.

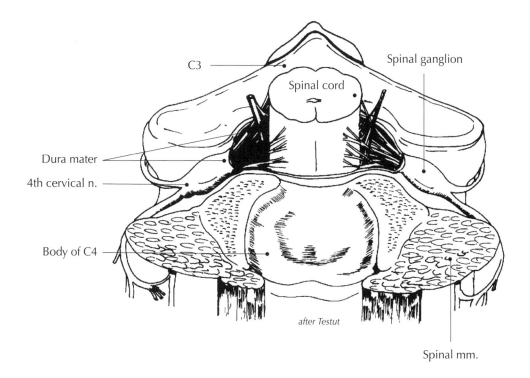

Fig. 5-3: Dura mater extension on the nerves

Bilateral inequality of dura mater tension

The dura mater is primarily extensible longitudinally, between the skull and the sacrum. However, our experience indicates that this longitudinal tension is usually not bilaterally equal, for the following reasons:

- one side is more flexible and mobile than the other. For example, right-handed people tend to pick up objects by bending down on the left side.
- fetal positioning leads to a relatively restricted side and a relatively free side
- various traumas accumulate to reinforce the original lateral dura mater stresses, or create new ones.

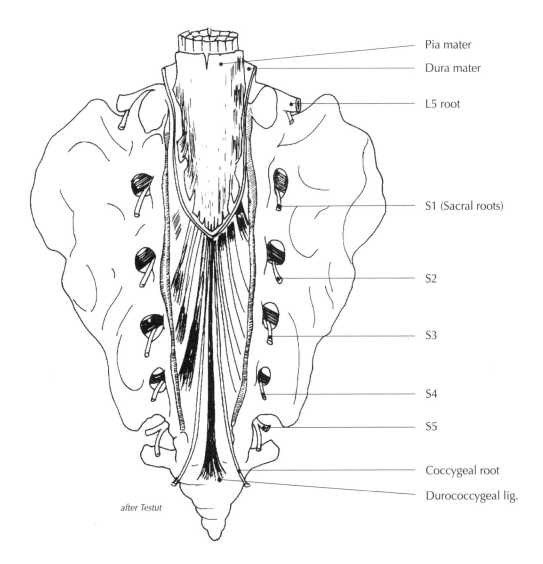

Fig. 5-4: Dural cul-de-sac
(posterior section of the sacrum has been removed)

It is therefore necessary to test the longitudinal tension of the dura both along its axis and laterally. Patients with increased dura mater tension on one side are more prone to ipsilateral problems such as cervicobrachial neuralgia and sciatica. Even without any obvious pathology, the cervicobrachial or lumbosacral nerve roots of the fixed dura mater side are under more tension and less stretchable.

Key points for dura mater evaluation

In evaluation and treatment of the dura mater there are a few key points where the dura mater is more easily restricted and where our techniques are most effective. They are:

- superior longitudinal and transverse sinuses
- occipitoatloid junction
- cervicobrachial plexus (at C4-C6)
- T8-T9
- lumbosacral plexus (especially the sciatic roots)
- sacrum and coccyx.

Dura mater restrictions

Dura mater restrictions of vertebral origin usually result from violent trauma to the cranium, spinal column, or sacrum. The dura mater is damaged by the hard bony tissues, and restrictions are caused by stretching and micro-tears.

Dura mater distensibility

Histologically, the dura mater is a resistant fibrous tissue whose purpose is to protect the brain and spinal cord. Because it is the container within which the CNS "floats," restrictions in the dura mater can cause increased CSF pressure. Furthermore, post-traumatic dural restrictions can produce epileptic seizures, vascular problems, headaches, dizziness, spinal pain, digestive dysfunction, genital pain, and many other problems, depending on the segmental level affected.

Listening tests

General listening

Stand behind the patient, who is in a seated or upright position. Place the palm of your dominant hand on the vertex of the head slightly behind the coronal suture, and allow the hand to be drawn naturally to the area with the greatest degree of restriction. The longitudinal axis of your hand matches that of the patient's skull *(Fig. 5-5)*. This important test is described in detail in Barral (1989).

In the case of a cranial dura mater restriction, your palm adheres rapidly but superficially to the skull. The hand remains essentially flat, with only slight sidebending, pronation, or supination, and slides toward the side of the restriction before being drawn to it.

Alternately, your hand can be placed transversely with the knuckles running along the longitudinal axis of the patient's skull. From this position your hand will only rock slightly one way or the other. Regardless of hand placement, general listening permits you to determine the existence of, and precisely locate, important areas of restriction.

Local listening

The patient is supine, legs extended, arms at rest at the sides. Seated behind the head, place the palm of your dominant hand behind the coronal suture, with the axis of your hand aligned with the longitudinal axis of the skull, and your index finger pointed toward the glabella. This position is optimal for analysis of dura mater restrictions, their location, extent, and relation to other restrictions, for example, those of the sutures *(Fig. 5-6 a & b)*.

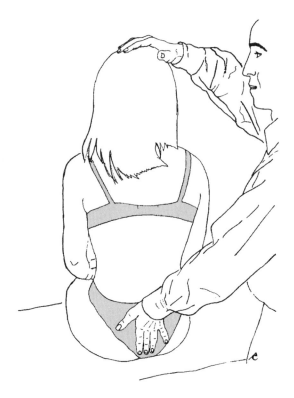

Fig. 5-5: General listening: seated position

When a dura mater restriction exists, your entire palm is drawn to it. Your hand glides superficially toward the problematic area, then is strongly attracted and rotates slightly toward the restriction. Your palm will stay relatively flat because dural restrictions affect an area of the dura, not merely a point. When listening reveals dural restrictions, your hand should not remain supinated or pronated. For spinal dura mater restrictions, your palm is drawn posteroinferiorly.

Sutural problems can be detected using the same test. For them, the pull will be rather superficial and can be easily tested. For example, if the palm is pulled anteriorly and laterally toward the right coronal suture, retest by placing the heel of your hand on the frontal bone, anterior to the coronal suture. If it is the suture which is pulling your hand, the pull will now be posterior and lateral.

When doing local listening to the skull, be wary when the pull appears to be deeper into the cranium. If the hand supinates or pronates and remains on its side, it is being attracted by a problem deeper inside the skull, such as a cyst or tumor. Diagnostic imaging is often appropriate for these patients.

Diagnosis of sutural restrictions

Our presentation here of cranial procedures is neither comprehensive nor revolutionary. For more information, we refer you to the eminent American and European writers in this important discipline: William Gartner Sutherland, Harold Magoun, John

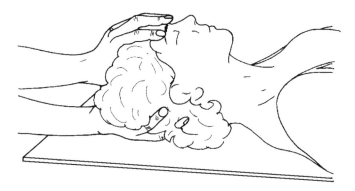

Fig. 5-6a: Dura mater diagnosis by local listening

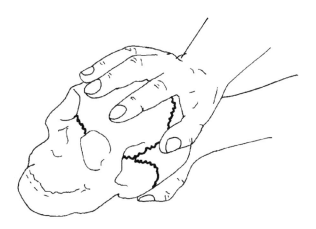

Fig. 5-6b: Local listening for the skull: hand placement

Upledger, Lionnelle Issartel, and Marc Bozetto. Here, we shall simply describe several structural manipulations which we have found to be effective following trauma, especially when combined with functional techniques. Many of these tests and manipulations focus on the cranial sutures *(Fig. 5-7)*.

General sutural tests

The skull has considerable sutural elasticity. With bilateral compression, the diameter of the cranium can be reduced by a centimeter. The bone, periosteum, and dura mater retain "memory." We like to evaluate general sutural cranial elasticity before evaluating individual sutures.

Sagittal examination of the skull

The subject is supine. Place one hand under the occiput and the other on the frontal. Be sure that your frontal hand is completely in front of the coronal suture. Compress the skull by pushing the frontal hand toward the occiput. The suboccipital

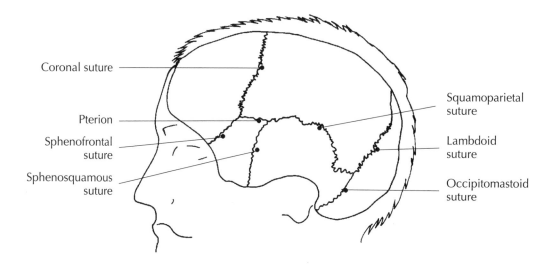

Coronal suture

Pterion

Sphenofrontal
suture

Sphenosquamous
suture

Squamoparietal
suture

Lambdoid
suture

Occipitomastoid
suture

Fig. 5-7: Cranial sutures (lateral view)

hand may remain passive, or actively help compression by moving toward the frontal *(Fig. 5-8)*. Active movement can be quite strong, yet should never cause any pain.

After shortening the sagittal diameter of the skull as described above, evaluate its return to normal position. A slow or difficult return indicates superior dura mater compression (along the sagittal sinus) or restriction of the falx. Difficulty in compression indicates a lack of osseous elasticity, with impaction of the coronal suture.

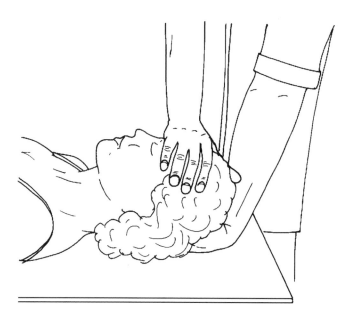

Fig. 5-8: Sagittal evaluation of the skull

Transverse examination of the skull

The patient is again supine, but with the head resting alternately on one side and then the other. For the left side, for example, the patient's head is rotated to the right. Place the palm of your left hand on the left frontoparietal region, and rest your right hand on the table, with the palm on the right frontoparietal region. Push the two hands toward each other, and evaluate the compression and return of the skull *(Fig. 5-9a)*. This can also be done with the hands reversed *(Fig. 5-9b)*. A difficult compression indicates an intra-osseous problem and restriction of the lateral sutures. A difficult return is more likely the sign of a lateral dura mater restriction.

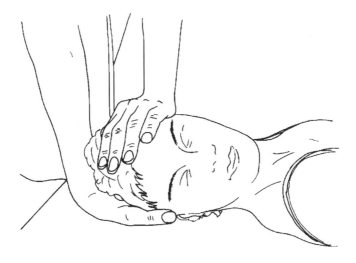

Fig. 5-9a: Transverse evaluation of the skull

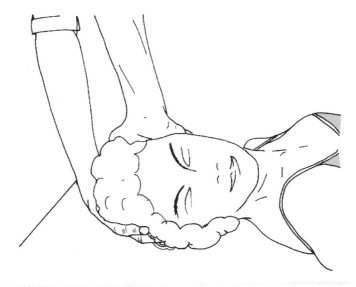

Fig. 5-9b: Transverse evaluation of the skull (hands reversed)

Test of the coronal suture

DIRECT

The patient is supine, legs extended, hands resting on the thorax. Sit behind the patient and place the palm of your dominant hand at the frontal level, immediately in front of the coronal suture, so that your middle finger is in the sagittal plane. The occiput rests on your other palm. Push the frontal anteriorly and slightly superiorly, as if you were trying to separate the two edges of the coronal suture *(Fig. 5-10)*. Start by pushing on the middle part, and then alternately the two lateral sections.

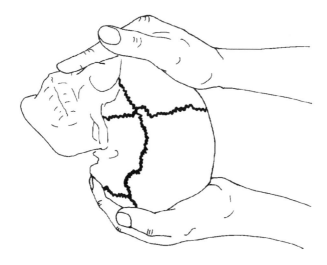

Fig. 5-10: Coronal suture test
(palm is in front of suture)

If there is a sutural restriction, you cannot feel the normal, slight sutural distensibility—it's as if you were testing a piece of wood. When discussing sutures, the term "mobility test" is inappropriate. *You feel distensibility, not mobility.* Sutures dampen stress, and permit a certain degree of *cranial deformability* as well as osseous elasticity. The coronal suture is rarely completely restricted, but we often see small restricted areas about 2cm long.

INDIRECT

Sutural tension is created by pushing the frontal anterosuperiorly, as above, but in the second phase you slightly release the pressure to let your palm do the listening. The listening test allows you to locate points of restriction much more precisely.

Other sutures

Other sutures (e.g., coronal, squamoparietal, lambdoid, occipitomastoid) may be evaluated by separation into two parts. Large restrictions are usually the result of cranial trauma or fetal malposition. We will give two examples here, but the same principles apply to any suture.

SQUAMOPARIETAL SUTURE

The subject is in lateral decubitus position, with the head resting on the side opposite the side being tested. Place the heel of one palm on the parietal to direct it superomedially, and the other on the temporal, to push it inferolaterally, as if you wanted to separate the two bones *(Fig. 5-11)*.

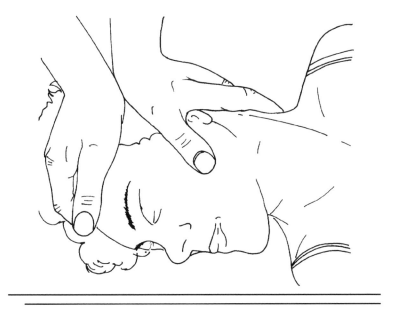

Fig. 5-11: Squamoparietal suture test

As in general sutural evaluation, your hands act with a certain amount of force, but never cause cranial or cervical pain. In addition to sutural distensibility, you should feel the osseous elasticity of the parietal and temporal bones themselves. This test can also be performed with listening.

OCCIPITOPETROSAL TEST

Schematically, we can envision the anterior part of the occiput (basilar and condylar sections) as forming a triangular structure, with its anterior point located between the two petrous pillars. Trauma-induced whiplash often causes unilateral or bilateral impaction of the occiput, which is forcefully pushed between the temporals. The force of the trauma is concentrated on the petrojugular suture, but also affects the petrobasilar and occipitomastoid sutures. The purpose of this test is to verify whether the occiput can be separated from the two petrous pillars, or if it is jammed.

With the subject supine, hold the head in your palms. Press the little fingers on the median occipital line, with the middle and ring fingers placed laterally on both sides. The pads of your fingers penetrate the tissues deeply and approach the posterior arc of the atlas as closely as possible *(Fig. 5-12)*.

Place your index finger directly behind the mastoid process and in front of the occipitomastoid suture.

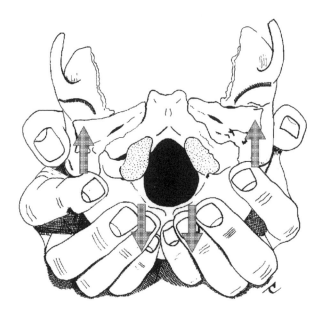

Fig. 5-12: Occipitopetrosal test

- Press the pads of the occipital fingers against the inferior part of the occipital ridges to get properly anchored.
- Using your index fingers, make a fixed point by maintaining the mastoid processes in an anterior direction.
- With your occipital hold, test the freedom of occipital disengagement between the temporals with a backward rotational movement.

If there is a restriction, the occiput cannot be moved freely between the temporals. If the restriction is bilateral, no sensation of movement is felt. If the restriction is unilateral, the difference in perception of movement between the free and fixed sides is obvious.

Membranous craniofacial system

During craniofacial trauma, membrane tensions do not always affect the sutures. There is a subtle articular play between the face and skull, which we term membranous, but is more accurately "osteosuturomyomembranous." If one of the components loses its distensibility, the skull slowly becomes restricted, rendering sutural manipulations alone ineffective.

The face has a lower density than the skull, and therefore a different response to trauma. Much of the force exerted on the face is transferred to the skull. It is important to evaluate and treat the face and its junctions with the skull in trauma patients.

Evaluation of palate

The patient is supine, arms at the sides, legs extended. Position yourself facing the patient's right shoulder *(Fig. 5-13)*. Always wear gloves when working around the mouth.

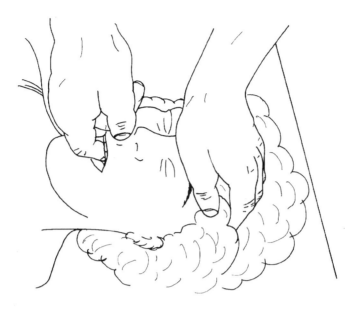

Fig. 5-13: Test of the palate

Median section

The anterior (hard) palate is of interest to us. Crook the index finger of your dominant hand and place its tip on the anterior part of the median palatine suture, immediately behind the incisive fossa *(Fig. 5-14)*.

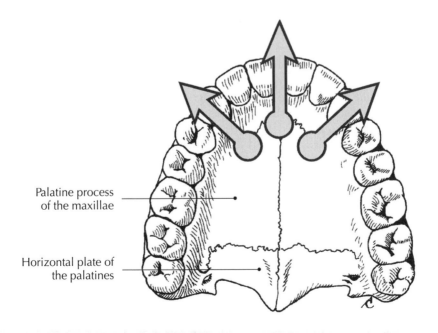

Palatine process
of the maxillae

Horizontal plate of
the palatines

Fig. 5-14: Support points during test of the palate

Exert traction anteriorly and slightly superiorly. If everything is free, you should feel distensibility and mobility of the bony palate relative to the cranium. If there is restriction of the palate or maxillae, you will not feel this slight movement; rather, you will have an impression of firmness and resistance which holds back the palate.

LATERAL SECTIONS

In the same position, place your index finger on either side of the median palatine suture, near the dental arch, between the canines and premolars. Move the crooked index finger anteriorly, laterally, and superiorly. Repeat on the other side.

Median palatine tension often indicates central sagittal dura mater tension involving the falx cerebri. Lateral palatine tension more frequently indicates dura mater restriction or lateral and posterior sutural restriction.

All these tests can be performed using listening. For this, you apply less tension through your fingers, and follow the listening into the restriction.

Maxillae and cranium

We are more interested in the connections of the maxillae with the skull than in the bones themselves. The maxillae have many interesting connections to the bones of the face and the base of the skull:

- *superiorly and laterally with the zygomatics.* There are two lateral pillars formed by the ascending portion of the maxillae, joined to the lateral orbital processes and also to the zygomatic arch. The connection of the maxillae to the cranium is primarily by these two pillars, which help split up the force in craniofacial trauma.
- *superiorly and medially with the nasal, lacrimal, and frontal bones.* The median pillar joining the face to the cranium is composed of the nasal and lacrimal bones, the frontal, and the two ascending frontal processes of the maxillae, joined to the internal orbital process.
- *posteriorly with the pterygoid process*
- *inferiorly with the opposite maxilla.*

Craniofacial membranous test

With the patient supine, place the thumb and index finger of the dominant hand on both sides of the maxilla (inside the mouth, lateral and superior to the teeth), at the root of the zygomatic processes. Between the thumb and middle finger (or the index finger for children) the other hand holds the frontal at the level of the temples, slightly above the sphenofrontal suture *(Figs. 5-15 & 5-16)*.

DIRECT TEST

Move both hands along the transverse plane and push the frontal toward one side and the maxillary toward the other. You should be able to feel true osteosutural membraneous elasticity. It should be equal on both sides, while in the case of a restriction, one side is flexible and the other is rigid. Remember, this is a gross motion; to appreciate it you need to use more than subtle forces.

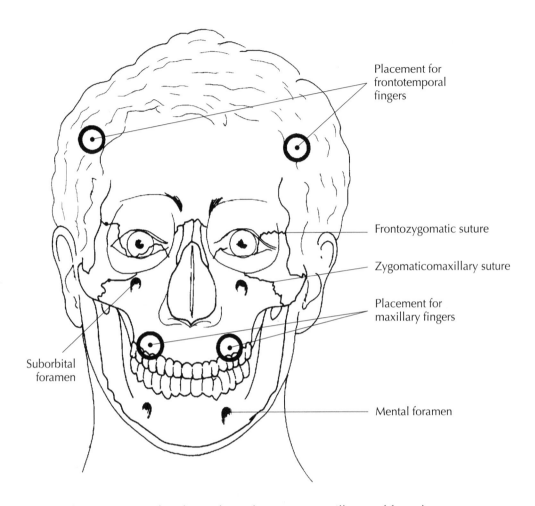

Fig. 5-15: Craniofacialsutural membrane test: maxillary and frontal support

INDIRECT TEST

In general, we prefer to perform craniofacial tests in the direction of the listening. This permits more subtle manipulation without risk of damage to the delicate craniofacial system.

Your position is the same as in the direct test. Instead of actively and laterally mobilizing the maxillae on the frontal or vice versa, let your hands follow the direction of the listening toward the side of the restriction. You should exaggerate the movement, as this induction is very active.

CONCLUSION

There are three possibilities, listed below.

- If you feel the maxilla go laterally, the problem is facial.
- If the frontal goes laterally, there is probably a cranial restriction.

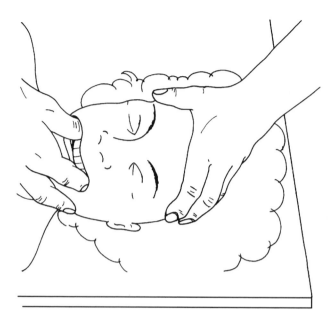

Fig. 5-16: Craniofacial membranous test

- If the two hands are drawn in opposite directions, there is craniofacial mechanical conflict, typically resulting from violent craniofacial trauma, intrauterine stress, or heavy-handed obstetrical maneuvers.

Direct tests evaluate overall craniofacial mobility. Listening permits us to distinguish among membranous, sutural, and intraosseous restrictions.

- Membranous restrictions always allow some room for movement.
- Sutural restrictions are felt as a hard restriction during movement.
- Intraosseous restrictions give an *immediate* impression of a barrier.

Among the symptoms of craniofacial restriction are headaches, sinus pain, sinusitis, tempomandibular dysfunction, and cervical pain.

Listening test for maxillae

In listening, your palm is drawn anteriorly toward the orbits, then laterally toward one of the maxillae. Pull is almost always toward the maxilla rather than the mandible. With positive maxillary listening, one often finds ipsilateral inflammation or cervical restriction.

Craniospinal dura mater tests

Suboccipital traction and listening (direct)

This traction test is useful for distinguishing occipitocranial, spinal, and lumbosacral restrictions of the dura mater. Traction combined with listening, which is less well-known, greatly increases the accuracy of the diagnosis.

The patient is supine, arms at the sides, and legs extended to increase dura mater tension. Seated behind the patient's head, place your palms under the occiput with the index finger of the non-dominant hand on the inferior occipital line, immediately above the atlas. Place the index finger of the dominant hand on the other index finger so that traction is not exerted directly on the occiput *(Fig. 5-17)*. After placing the index fingers on the center of the inferior occipital line, place them to the right and to the left. This allows you to test both the central and lateral sections of the dura mater. Alternatively, you can place the middle finger of your dominant hand in the midline of the inferior occipital line, with an index finger or either side.

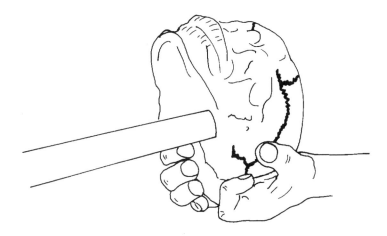

Fig. 5-17: Listening with traction on the cylinder of the dura mater

Be alert for small suboccipital nodes, which are common during puberty and indicate subclinical infectious problems (involving the teeth, throat, ear, or nose) or generalized fatigue. Do not place the index finger directly on these nodes; this would create irritation, which renders your diagnosis and treatment ineffective.

Occipitocranial test (indirect)

Place an index finger between the occiput and atlas and perform listening. The finger will be drawn in a superior direction for cranial dura mater problems, or an inferior direction for spinal dura mater problems.

Occipital traction test for spinal dura mater

Perform this test only during the craniosacral expansion phase. As soon as you feel the craniosacral expansion, exert traction on the occiput longitudinally in a superior direction. Be careful! This test will be imprecise at best and difficult to interpret if you exert traction during the craniosacral relaxation phase.

Next, slightly relax the traction and allow your index finger to be drawn in the direction of listening. Close your eyes to achieve total concentration. You should feel actual dura mater elongation with a strong sense of gliding. Diagnoses are as follows.

- *Immediate resistance to traction* indicates either general restriction of the entire dura mater (following major trauma), or a significant restriction of C1. In the latter case, we feel immediate resistance, and a secondary impression of dura mater distensibility underlying vertebral restriction.
- *An initial sensation of distensibility*, followed immediately by resistance to stretching, signifies a restriction of the vertebra and dura mater located lower down.
- *Lateral resistance to traction* usually signifies interapophyseal, costovertebral, rib, or radicular restriction. In this case, the test is done with lateral displacement of the finger under the occiput, to the side of the restriction. Traction/listening is performed again on the longitudinal side to localize the problem.
- Post-traumatic or intrauterine restrictions of the dura mater often *limit longitudinal dura mater distensibility*, both centrally and laterally.

We must emphasize that traction/listening is very different from simple traction. The movement accomplished in the space appears to have a greater amplitude. With your eyes closed, you have the impression that traction in the cranial expansion phase is practically limitless. The dura mater seems to glide slowly and harmoniously in the direction of your index finger.

Occiput-sacrum traction test for spinal dura mater

The patient is supine. Place one hand under the occiput and the other under the sacrum.

The occipital hand approaches the occiput contralaterally, in forced pronation, to benefit from support of the back of the hand on the table. The fingers are directed toward the vertex, adhering as closely as possible to the cranial axis of symmetry. The sacral hand also respects the symmetry of the bone. The middle finger is on the median axis, index and ring finger on the sacral base, thumb and little finger on the iliac bone. The inferolateral angles of the sacrum rest on the base of the thenar and hypothenar eminences *(Fig. 5-18)*.

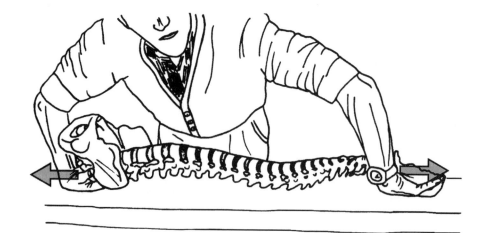

Fig. 5-18: Test of the two extremities of the spinal dura mater

Make a slight effort to move the two hands apart, as if attempting to slide the occiput superiorly and the sacrum inferiorly. The occipital and sacral bony insertions act as levers, mobilizing the membranous structures. You can appreciate the subtle elasticity of these structures and their freedom to slide into the epidural space.

Superior cranial dura mater

We should evaluate the superior cranial dura mater following direct cranial trauma, that is, when the patient has fallen on the head or been hit on the head by a heavy object, as well as in cases of intrauterine fetal stress or scoliosis. The upper part of the dura mater follows exactly the direction of the longitudinal sinus.

Test of the longitudinal sinus

The longitudinal sinus is located deep within the dura mater, occupying the convex edge of the falx cerebri. It is the largest of the sinuses (30-40cm long), and the most exposed to trauma. It begins in front of the crista galli and extends to the internal occipital protuberance, where it contributes to the confluence of sinuses. It gradually increases in size as it goes posteriorly. Two lateral sinuses emerge from the confluence of sinuses. Their direction serves as a basis for lateral testing of the dura mater *(Figs. 5-19 & 5-20)*.

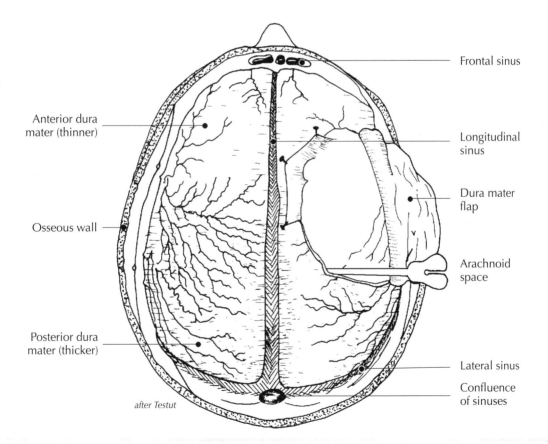

Fig. 5-19: Dura mater and venous sinus

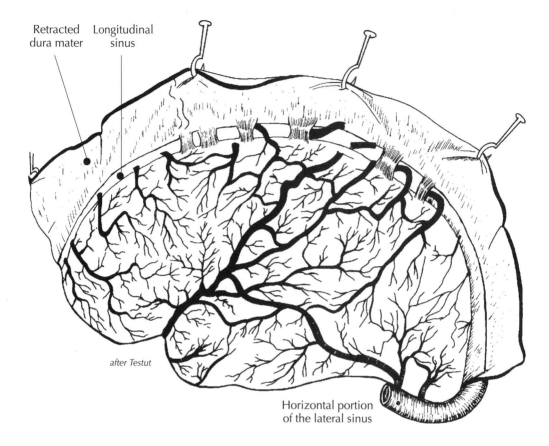

Retracted
dura mater

Longitudinal
sinus

after Testut

Horizontal portion
of the lateral sinus

Fig. 5-20: Relationship of the dura mater to the longitudinal and lateral sinuses

For the test, the patient is supine, legs extended, hands on the chest. Place the hypothenar eminence of your dominant hand behind the coronal suture, with your middle finger along the axis of the sagittal suture. The patient's occiput rests on your other hand *(Fig. 5-21)*.

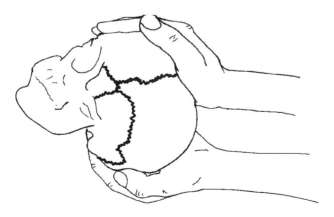

Fig. 5-21: Superior longitudinal sinus test

The *direct test* consists of pushing the palm of the dominant hand anteroinferiorly. When the superior dura mater is free, you should feel distensibility and a return to normal. Movement of your palm should be strong, yet not cause any discomfort or pain.

For the *indirect test*, slightly relax the pressure behind the coronal suture to allow your hand to be drawn into listening. This test yields more precise information on which section of the longitudinal sinus to treat. The middle and posterior sections are the most commonly restricted.

Posterior cranial dura mater

Tests and manipulations of the posterior cranial dura mater are based on the direction of the two lateral cranial sinuses, to which it is closely linked.

Lateral sinuses

These two cranial sinuses are 10-15mm wide. They begin at the level of the internal protuberance (confluence of sinuses) and end at the level of the posterior foramen lacerum where the internal jugular vein is formed. *The continuity with this vein explains why thoracic inhalation can be felt through the lateral sinus.*

Note: Manipulation of the cervicothoracic inlet is important for cranial venous circulation. It helps restore negative intravenous pressure for optimal cranial blood circulation. The same principle applies to the vertebral veins. Any injury to the superior part of the dura mater has repercussions on the general cranial venous system.

The lateral sinus receives blood from the posterior cerebellar veins, inferior and posterior cerebral veins, and mastoid veins.

The horizontal portion of the lateral sinus belongs to the neck region. Superficially, it corresponds:

- posteriorly, to the superior line of the occiput
- anteriorly, to the parietomastoid suture.

A line drawn from the superior edge of the auditory meatus to the external occipital protuberance demarcates it well. This portion of the sinus is concave in the large circumference of the tentorium cerebelli, which is always involved in testing and manipulation of this area.

The descending portion of the lateral sinus runs from the internal occipital protuberance to the posterosuperior angle of the mastoid. It then bends in a right angle and ends up in the posterior foramen lacerum.

Occipitomastoid test of the lateral sinus

DIRECT TEST

The patient is in lateral decubitus position, head turned toward the side opposite the occipitomastoid region being tested. Standing behind the patient, with your elbows flexed, place the palm of your dominant hand against the posterior edge of the mastoid and push it anteriorly and laterally *(Fig. 5-22)*. This stretches the descending portion of the lateral sinus *(Fig. 5-23)*. The other palm presses between the internal occipital protuberance and the parietal to create an active counter-support.

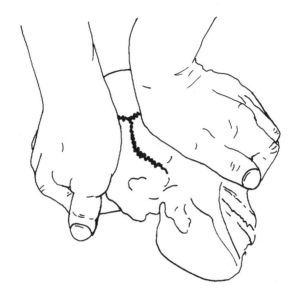

Fig. 5-22: Occipitomastoid test

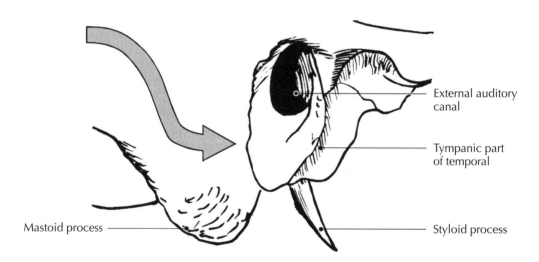

External auditory canal

Tympanic part of temporal

Mastoid process

Styloid process

Fig. 5-23: Direction of the lateral sinus, to be followed during the test of the posterior dura mater

The cervical column should not be involved in (i.e., irritated by) the movements you perform. Concentrate the stretching specifically on the skull. This test includes the occipitomastoid suture. Always evaluate differences in distensibility between the two sides.

INDIRECT TEST

Slightly relax the pressure on the descending position of the lateral sinus, allowing your hand to be drawn into listening in the direction of a possible restriction.

Cervicobrachial plexus

Cervical plexus

This is the series of anastomoses formed by the anterior branches of the first four cervical nerves, before their peripheral division. Our test deals mainly with the deep descending branches of the third and fourth cervical nerves. The anterior branches occupy the groove formed by the superior surface of the transverse processes, and pass between the two intertransverse muscles behind the vertebral artery.

The cervical plexus is situated behind the posterior edge of the sternocleidomastoid, deep to the internal jugular vein, internal carotid artery, and vagus nerve. It anastomoses with the hypoglossus, vagus, and sympathetic nerves.

Phrenic nerve

This paired nerve arises from the fourth cervical and from branches the third and fifth cervical nerves. It descends on the anterior surface of the anterior scalene muscle. At the entry to the thorax, the phrenic passes between the subclavian artery and vein. The left phrenic descends behind the brachiocephalic venous trunk, parallel to the subclavian artery.

Brachial plexus

This is formed by the anterior branches of the last four cervical and the first thoracic nerve before they begin their peripheral distribution. The brachial plexus traverses the subclavian triangle at its posteroinferior section, where it rests on the posterior scalene. It is covered by the omohyoid muscle and the middle and deep cervical aponeuroses. Behind the clavicle it is separated by the subclavian muscle. It rests on the first rib and the superior digitation of the serratus anterior. It is behind the pectoral muscles, anterior to the subscapular tendon, and between the two scalenes. The subclavian artery is found at the lower section of the plexus, slightly anterior to it *(Fig. 5-24)*.

Test of the cervicobrachial plexus

Irritation of the nerve roots surrounded by the perineurium, an extension of the dura mater, can laterally destabilize the spinal dura mater. The opposite is also true, that is, abnormal lateral tension of the spinal dura mater promotes irritation and compression of the cervical or brachial plexus. This test permits you to determine the precise location of proximal foraminal irritation and distal nerve inflammation.

DIRECT TEST

The patient is supine, legs extended, arms at the sides.

Step one: Seated behind the patient's head, use your contralateral hand to support the neck. For example, for the right cervicobrachial plexus, place the slightly crooked middle or index finger of your left hand on the anterolateral sections of the edges and behind the right intertransverse spaces. Push your finger anteriorly, between the interlamellar spaces, until you find a little bump or indentation which is sensitive, and sometimes painful *(Fig. 5-25)*.

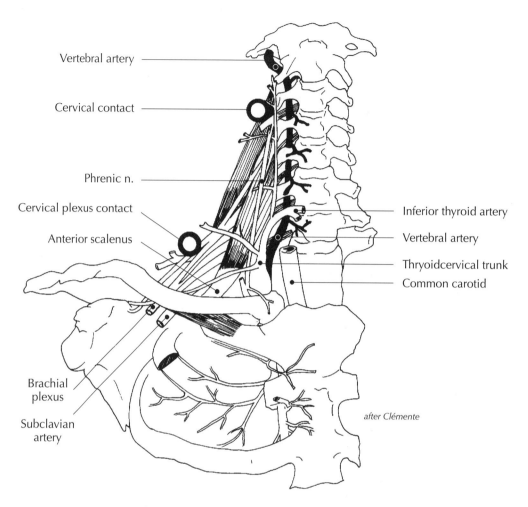

Vertebral artery

Cervical contact

Phrenic n.

Cervical plexus contact

Anterior scalenus

Inferior thyroid artery

Vertebral artery

Thryoidcervical trunk

Common carotid

Brachial plexus

Subclavian artery

after Clémente

Fig. 5-24: Regional anatomy of the cervicobrachial plexus

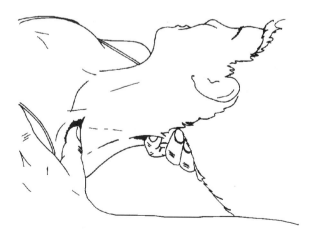

Fig. 5-25: Cervicobrachial plexus test

Step two: Use the thumb of your other hand to seek out sensitive areas. These are usually located at either:

- the space between the anterolateral trapezius and the lateral clavicle
- the space between the medial clavicle and the anterior scalene.

The second of these is more common and can be found fairly easily by first locating the subclavian artery and then feeling slightly posterolaterally. The palm of your hand should encompass the lateral trapezius and the posterior glenohumoral joint. With your thumb, seek out the indented and sensitive zones within this space.

Step three: Once you have your fingers on the right areas, try to connect them, stretching the distal section anteriorly and laterally. You know that you have found the connection when you feel an increase in cervical tension, by stretching the lateral hardened zone. Make careful note of where the tension is, and where it seems to be going.

INDIRECT TEST

In this test, listening is indispensable to refine your location of the areas of restriction and to link them together. Treatment will be effective only if this connection is made. You can also use manual thermal diagnosis to find localized conflict zones, since they radiate heat.

Sacral dura mater test

A dura mater, sacral, or sacrococcygeal restriction gives a limited suboccipital longitudinal traction test at the end of stretching. It is as if the dura mater were held down by a weight at the end of movement. Try to corroborate this test by a more localized test, changing the zones of support depending upon whether the restrictions are anterior or posterior.

Test for anterior restrictions

The patient is seated on the exam table, hands crossed over the chest or behind the neck. Standing behind the patient, with your right foot braced on the table, support the patient, either by surrounding the shoulders, or (if the hands are behind the neck) by holding both elbows with your right hand.

Place your left hand anteriorly under the sacrum, so as to grasp the coccyx, sacrococcygeal joint, and part of the sacrum with your index finger and palm. Draw the sacrum and coccyx posteriorly and slightly inferiorly, to perform flexion of the sacral promontory (*Fig. 5-26*).

In the event of sacroiliac restriction, you will have an immediate impression of firmness, from the beginning of movement. Anterior dura mater tension is manifested by very restrained movement, as if there were a membranous brake.

Test for posterior restrictions

The patient is in the same position as above, with both hands behind the neck. Seated at the right or behind the patient, with your right foot resting on the table, support both elbows with your forearms.

Push the entire vertebral column into flexion. With the palm of your left hand, push the sacrum anteriorly at the beginning and end of the movement, as if you wanted to increase the posterior angle between L5 and S1.

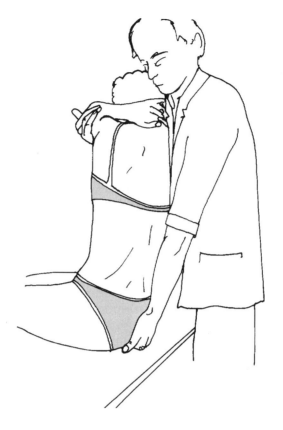

Fig. 5-26: Sacral dura mater test (seated position)

An anterior sacroiliac restriction is manifested by an absence of mobility from the beginning of movement. A dura mater restriction manifests as difficulty in drawing the sacrum anteriorly, and restrained movement.

Sciatic nerve

The *lumbosacral plexus* is the complex of nerves formed by the anterior branches of the last lumbar and first sacral pairs, before their peripheral distribution *(Fig. 5-27)*.

The *sciatic nerve* is the longest nerve in the human body. Its connections with the lumbosacral plexus enable us to affect the dura mater through the radicular perineurium.

In patients suffering from sciatica, more interest is usually paid to disco-radicular conflict than to the nerve itself. However, by stretching the sciatic nerve, we can treat inflammation of its roots, and restriction of the normally mobile radicular sleeve and the epidural and foraminal veins.

After certain types of trauma, the dura mater is longitudinally restricted on one side. Even with lateral head or neck pain, it is useful to relax lateral tension of the dura mater at the level of the lumbosacral plexus. The superior attachments affect the lower attachments, and vice versa.

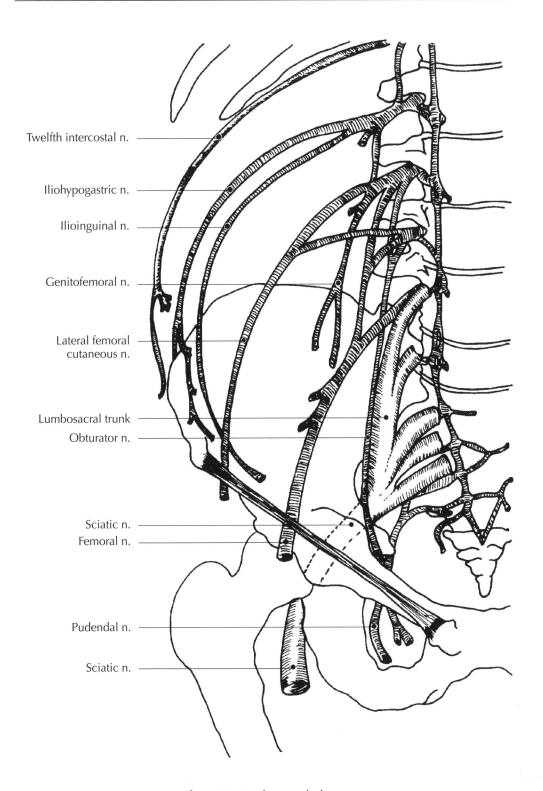

Twelfth intercostal n.

Iliohypogastric n.

Ilioinguinal n.

Genitofemoral n.

Lateral femoral
cutaneous n.

Lumbosacral trunk

Obturator n.

Sciatic n.

Femoral n.

Pudendal n.

Sciatic n.

Fig. 5-27: Lumbosacral plexus

Sciatic pathway and relationships

The nerve exits via the lower part of the greater sciatic notch and descends in the ischiofemoral groove, located between the ischial tuberosity and greater trochanter.

The sciatic nerve is covered by the piriformis muscle until the middle of the buttock, and by the inferior fasciculi of the gluteus maximus. The lesser sciatic is located behind it. Anteriorly it rests, from top to bottom, on the superior gemellus muscle, tendon of the internal obturator, inferior gemellus, and quadratus femoris *(Fig. 5-28)*.

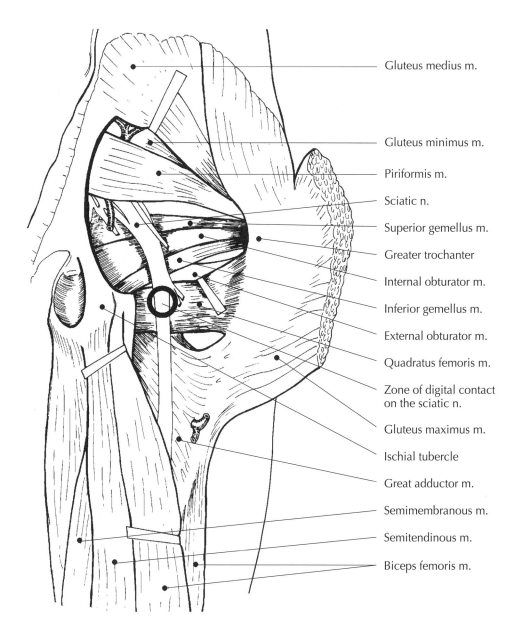

Gluteus medius m.

Gluteus minimus m.

Piriformis m.

Sciatic n.

Superior gemellus m.

Greater trochanter

Internal obturator m.

Inferior gemellus m.

External obturator m.

Quadratus femoris m.

Zone of digital contact on the sciatic n.

Gluteus maximus m.

Ischial tubercle

Great adductor m.

Semimembranous m.

Semitendinous m.

Biceps femoris m.

Fig. 5-28: Sciatic nerve (ischiotrochanter approach)

Stretching test of the sciatic nerve

The patient is supine, both hands on the abdomen, knee flexed on the side to be tested, other knee extended. You sit on the table, in front of the side to be tested.

For the right sciatic nerve, place the index finger of the left hand, flattened, in the ischiofemoral groove. This groove is flexible under your fingers. Draw your index finger in a superior direction, until you feel the firm transverse zone comprised of the lower edge of the piriformis. Next, gently move the finger in an inferior direction to feel the longitudinal "cord" formed by the sciatic nerve. This small cord is difficult to find in pain-free subjects, but is easier in sciatica patients because the mechanical tension of the sciatic nerve is more intense.

Place the palm of your right hand on the anterolateral part of the knee on the treated side. Flex the thigh while abducting and sidebending the hip, to permit positioning your left index finger higher up and more deeply in the ischiofemoral groove.

First method: Once you have located the tension in the sciatic nerve, abduct, medially rotate, and extend the leg, while pressing the sciatic nerve in the ischiofemoral groove *(Fig. 5-29).* The extension of the lower leg enables you to stretch the sciatic nerve. It is difficult to stretch the sciatic nerve inferiorly when treating a sacral dura mater restriction.

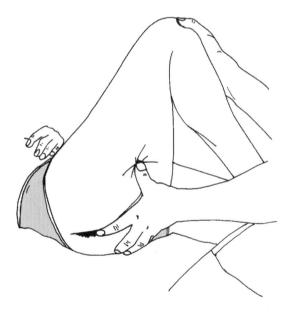

Fig. 5-29: Stretching test of the sciatic nerve (first method)

Despite its difficulty to perform, we strongly recommend this test. It enables you to find and treat restrictions of the radicular sleeve. If mobilization of the lower leg is difficult because of the patient's size or weight, try another method.

Second method: Position the patient's leg in abduction or external rotation by placing the foot on the medial surface of the nontreated thigh. Ask the patient to slide the leg on the table along the entire length of the lower leg, until the two legs are stretched out together.

Place your two index fingers next to each other, and press the superior finger firmly against the sciatic nerve to keep it in its compartment *(Fig. 5-30)*.

Use listening to let your finger be drawn to the area of tension. With practice, you can determine exactly where tension in the sciatic nerve is greatest (usually laterally).

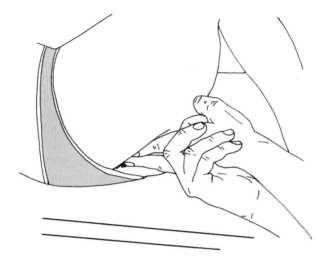

Fig. 5-30: Stretching test of the sciatic nerve (second method)

Tests of hip rotator muscles

Stretching of the lateral rotators of the hip, either directly or indirectly, permits release of the sacrum and lumbosacral plexus as well as the dura mater. Several muscles and ligaments are involved *(Fig. 5-31)*.

Each attachment of the hip, through the membranous tension it creates, affects these lateral rotator muscles, and through them, the sciatic nerve. Our colleagues Didier Prat and Louis Rommevaux, who have done considerable work in this area, emphasize the unique relationship between the bladder and obturator membrane. Any abnormal mechanical tension of the hip can destabilize the delicate muscular/membranous equilibrium of the bladder.

Piriformis muscle

This arises from the anterior surface of the sacrum at the level of S2-S4, and from several sites on the anterior surface of the sacrotuberous ligament. It passes through the greater sciatic notch and inserts on the trochanteric fossa *(Fig. 5-32)*. In the greater sciatic notch, it is closely related to the greater and lesser sciatic nerves.

Gemellus muscles

The superior and inferior gemellus originate respectively from the posterior surface of the sciatic spine and the superior part of the ischial tuberosity. Together they form a groove for the internal obturator, and rejoin at its distal end in a common tendon which inserts on the trochanteric fossa.

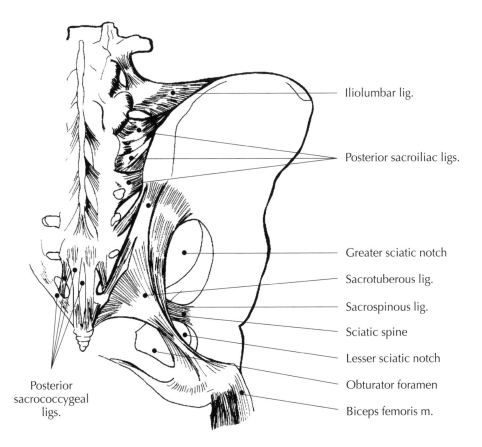

Iliolumbar lig.

Posterior sacroiliac ligs.

Greater sciatic notch

Sacrotuberous lig.

Sacrospinous lig.

Sciatic spine

Lesser sciatic notch

Obturator foramen

Biceps femoris m.

Posterior
sacrococcygeal
ligs.

Fig. 5-31: Ligaments of the pelvis

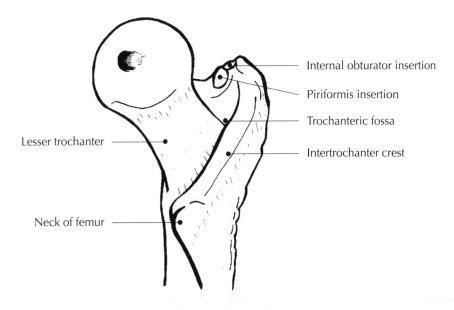

Internal obturator insertion

Piriformis insertion

Trochanteric fossa

Intertrochanter crest

Lesser trochanter

Neck of femur

Fig. 5-32: Trochanteric fossa of femur

Internal obturator muscle

This originates from the internal surface of the obturator membrane, inferior ramus of pubis, ramus of ischium, obturator fossa, and sciatic spine. It inserts on the greater trochanter. The aponeurosis of its posterior surface merges with the pelvic aponeurosis into which the medial fibers of the levator ani muscle are inserted.

External obturator muscle

It originates from the obturator membrane, pubis, and ascending ramus of the ischium. It runs laterally, obliquely along the posterior surface of the hip joint, and inserts on the trochanteric fossa.

Arcuate pubic ligament

This is not a lateral rotator muscle, but is very important for the interaction between the joint and muscles of the hip. It is a fibrous lamina (also known as the tendinous arch) consisting of the reinforced external portion of the obturator membrane. It is attached to the transverse ligament on the acetabulum and terminates above the spine of the pubis. The external obturator muscle has one of its origins from the arcuate pubic ligament *(Fig. 5-33)*.

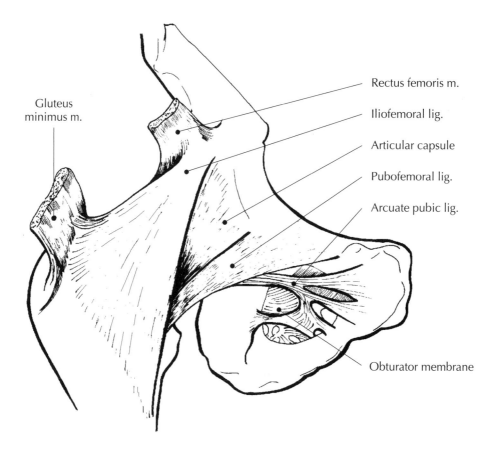

Fig. 5-33: Obturator membrane and hip ligaments

Quadratus femoris muscle

This arises from the lateral edge of the ischial tuberosity and inserts on the quadrate tubercle of the femur, near the greater trochanter.

Testing the lateral rotators

The subject is supine, hands crossed over the chest, leg on the tested side flexed, other leg extended. At the beginning, the position is the same as for stretching the sciatic nerve. You are seated on a stool facing the hip joint to be tested.

STEP ONE

For the muscles which insert on the trochanteric fossa, place the fingers of one hand on the intertrochanteric line, past the lateral part of the greater trochanter. Slide your fingers in the direction of the fossa, keeping them flat to avoid irritating the gluteal muscles or causing any painful contact in this sensitive region *(Fig. 5-34)*.

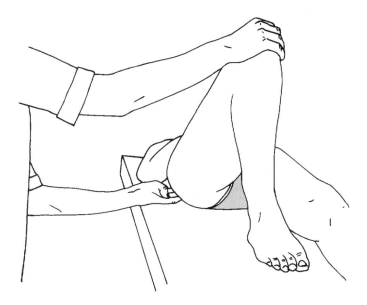

Fig. 5-34: Test of external rotators of the hip

STEP TWO

First method: The other hand holds the anterior surface of the knee and draws the leg in flexion and abduction. Take advantage of this movement to improve the position of your fingers in the trochanteric fossa. Stretch the greater trochanter backward and in slight sidebending at the beginning of the movement. Continue to stretch it inferiorly, posteriorly, and slightly laterally until you complete abduction/external rotation of the leg. Gradually draw the thigh into adduction/internal rotation and extension until the lower leg is resting on the table. At the end of the movement, it is important to maintain and increase external rotation of the thigh.

This test permits evaluation of the distensibility and elasticity of the lateral rotator muscles. It is considered to be positive if stretching of the muscles causes great sensitivity or pain, or if movement is limited. The two sides must be compared to objectively determine limitation of mobility.

Second method: This method may be preferable if the patient is heavy or large. Position the leg in abduction/external rotation, with the medial aspect of the foot resting on the medial surface of the opposite thigh. Ask the patient to slide the foot slowly along the length of the opposite lower leg until it is resting on the table.

During this time, stretch the greater trochanter with both hands laterally, inferiorly, and anteriorly at the beginning of the movement, then medially and posteriorly at the end. This enables you to increase the traction exerted by your hands on the femur.

Ischiofemoral test

This test allows evaluation of many structures, including the sacrotuberous and sacrospinal ligaments, perineum and its muscles (e.g., levator ani), lateral rotators of the hip, and the ischiofemoral ligament. The patient is in the same position as for the lateral rotator test described above, with the leg flexed on the side to be tested.

Stand facing the greater trochanter. For the right side, place the fingers of your right hand on the anteromedial part of the ischiopubic ramus, and hold it firmly. With your left hand on the lateral part of the bent knee, draw the femur in maximal adduction *(Fig. 5-35).*

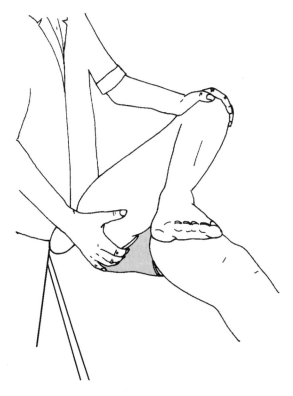

Fig. 5-35: Ischiofemoral test

Complete femoral adduction draws the ipsilateral ischium in abduction and slight sidebending. Move the right hand to draw the ischiopubic ramus toward you, and evaluate local fibromuscular distensibility and elasticity. Compare the two sides to determine which side is restricted. Experiment with femoral flexion to determine whether the restriction is more cephalad or caudad.

Diagnosis of traumatic pelvic restrictions

Tests of the sacral base

KNEE-RAISING TEST

The patient leans against a wall or piece of furniture, supported by the arms, which are extended and form a 90 degree angle with the thorax. Ask her to lift the flexed knee several times on each side, with more than 90 degrees of hip flexion. During this movement, place the tip of your thumbs on the posterosuperior sacral spines, then on the sacral base, and finally under the inferolateral sacral angles *(Fig. 5-36)*.

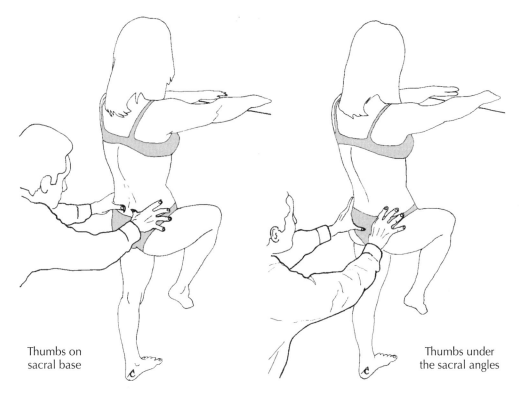

Thumbs on sacral base

Thumbs under the sacral angles

Fig. 5-36: Knee-raising test

The ilium becomes more posterior on the side of the bent knee, causing the sacrum to become laterally inclined on the side of the support leg. Compare the mobility of healthy subjects to that of patients with pelvic restrictions. With practice, the restrictions will become easier to detect.

TEST OF SACRAL COMPRESSION IN PRONE POSITION

We discussed this test in our book on urogenital manipulation (Barral, 1993). It permits evaluation of the role played by the uterosacral ligaments and uterine attachments in sacroiliac restriction.

The subject is supine. Place your hands on the posterior surface of the sacrum and compress it between the ilia in the direction of the pubic symphysis *(Fig. 5-37)*.

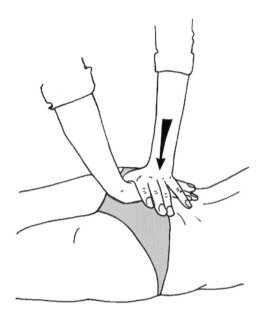

Fig. 5-37: Sacral compression

Note the quality of the compression, and of decompression when the sacrum returns to its original position. Compression and decompression are smooth and easy in a normal subject. In cases of post-traumatic pelvic restriction, compression is difficult or impossible at first on the side of the affected sacroiliac joint. When the decompression stage is slow or ratchety, especially on one side, it is usually due to a restriction or tear of a uterosacral ligament.

TEST OF SACRAL DECOMPRESSION

This test permits evaluation of restriction of the sacroiliac joints, and to a lesser extent, the lumbosacral and sacrococcygeal joints. It is directed primarily to the "joint" level, not the "tissue" level.

The patient is supine. Standing to her right, slide your right hand under the sacrum, with their longitudinal axes aligned. Place your left forearm on the right anterosuperior iliac spine, with your fingertips on the left anterosuperior iliac spine *(Fig. 5-38)*.

Tighten your support against the sacrum and lift it toward the ceiling, as if you wished to adjust it between the two iliac bones. With your upper right arm and left hand,

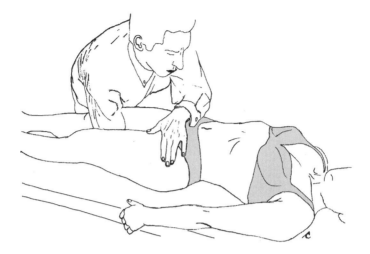

Fig. 5-38: Sacral decompression

separate the anterosuperior iliac spines from one another by pushing each one laterally. This movement permits extension of the powerful posterior sacroiliac ligamentous system *(Fig. 5-39)*.

This is a test of tissue elasticity. In normal subjects, the lifting of the sacrum is easily accomplished. You should feel definite movement without interference. If the lifting is difficult or uneven, there are sacral restrictions.

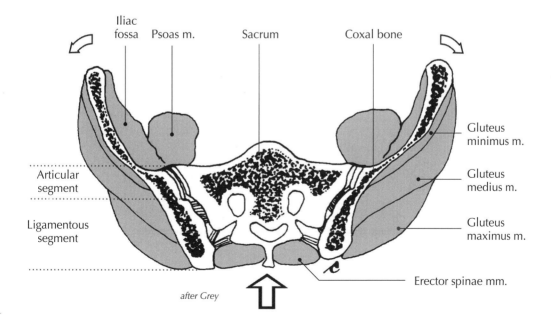

Fig. 5-39: Test of sacral decompression: horizontal section designed to demonstrate the two segments of the sacroiliac articulations

Interpretation

With a sacroiliac restriction, the iliac is depressed only on the free side, and the sacrum seems to rotate toward the restricted side. With some practice, this test will enable you to uncover an L5/ S1 restriction. You will feel a recess in the apical part of the sacrum, while the basal part remains joined to L5.

Once you have lifted the sacrum, you can further refine your interpretation by performing small movements of rotation and sidebending of the sacrum between the ilia.

Testing of the sacrum

The physiology of sacroiliac movements has been well-documented by our colleague Fred L. Mitchell, Jr. (1979). Concepts of anterior/posterior torsion and sacral flexion/extension are well-integrated and accepted in osteopathic practice. The difficulty arises in defining a specifically post-traumatic sacroiliac joint restriction. Trauma does not follow specific rules, and its effects on joints are unpredictable. However, in this case, we can distinguish two major classes of injury:

- post-traumatic sacral restrictions in sidebending *(Fig. 5-40)*; the differential diagnosis is superior movement of the ilium
- post-traumatic sacral restrictions in rotation *(Fig. 5-41)*; the differential diagnosis is anterior movement of the ilium.

Such restrictions may seem impossible in view of normal function of the sacroiliac joint. However, following trauma the sacrum is almost always fixed according to the above two classes of injury.

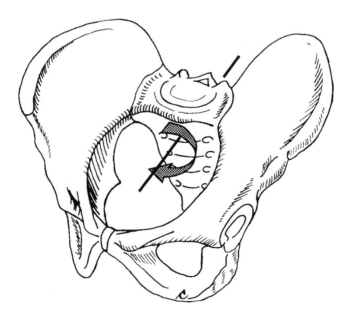

Fig. 5-40: Post-traumatic restriction of the sacrum in sidebending

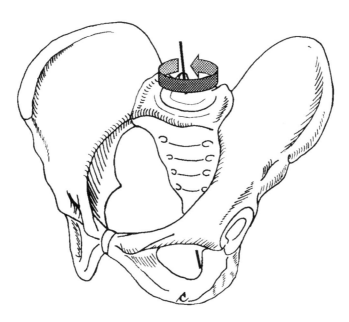

Fig. 5-41: Post-traumatic restriction of the sacrum in rotation

In our research, we came upon an article written by Strachan in 1939, describing sacral mobility in terms of these parameters of rotation and sidebending. In addition to supporting our point of view, his article demonstrates how well some authors understood the concept of loss of sacroiliac mobility well before Mitchell's codification (1954).

Post-traumatic sacral restrictions are easily diagnosed by the sacral compression and the knee-raising tests, as follows.

POST-TRAUMATIC RESTRICTION IN SIDEBENDING

- Sacral decompression test in prone position: upon compression, the sacrum is compressed between the ilia. At the end of the compression, slight resistance is felt at the recess between the ilia on the fixed side.
- Sacral decompression test in supine position: the sacrum tolerates decompression less on the fixed side, and seems to rotate to this side.
- Knee-raising test with your thumbs under the inferolateral sacral angles: there is normally sidebending of the sacrum toward the side of the supporting leg. If sacral sidebending does not occur, the diagnosis is post-traumatic sacral restriction in sidebending on the side of the raised leg.

POST-TRAUMATIC RESTRICTION IN ROTATION

- Sacral compression test in supine position: from the beginning, the sacrum resists compression between the ilia on the fixed side, while it compresses freely on the other side.
- Sacral decompression test in supine position: the sacrum clearly resists decompression on the fixed side, and seems stuck in rotation ipsilaterally.

- Knee-raising test with your thumbs on the sacral base inside the posterosuperior iliac spines: the sacrum normally rotates toward the side of the supporting leg. If this does not occur, the diagnosis is post-traumatic sacral restriction in rotation on the side of the raised leg.

These two lesion parameters frequently occur together, but one often predominates. Most often the side of the fixed sacroiliac is the side with the inferolateral angle of the sacrum down, or the side of the sacral base in a posterior position.

Examination of the coxal bone

Viewed from their sacroiliac surface, pelvic post-traumatic restrictions are well in line with conventional osteopathic teachings (Mitchell, 1979). We frequently find restrictions of the "upslipped" iliac type, as well as ilia in posterior or (less frequently) anterior rotation. In the last case we are referring to post-traumatic restriction rather than adaptation to unequal leg length, which can also cause anterior protrusion of the ilium. In adaptation (sometimes called first degree restriction), a small amount of movement persists. In post-traumatic restriction (second degree), all mobility is lost.

Examination of the coccyx

This examination should never be done in a haphazard or improvised manner. If the coccyx is restricted by tension from a myofascial chain, certain external techniques may be effective. In cases of post-traumatic restriction, only internal techniques are effective.

It is important to be able to decide when the coccyx requires internal (intrarectal) manipulation. This is a question frequently asked by novices. We use the test of mobility, in seated position, to evaluate axial compression, and sacrococcygeal flexion and sidebending (Fig. 5-42). The results of this test enable us to make the proper decision.

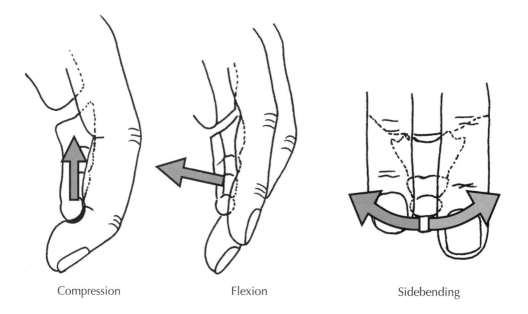

Compression   Flexion   Sidebending

Fig. 5-42: Tests of coccygeal mobility

We advise students to use a checklist of symptoms potentially revealed by the test:

- sensitive or painful axial compression
- sensitive or painful sacrococcygeal flexion
- restricted sacrococcygeal flexion
- sensitive or painful right sacrococcygeal sidebending
- restricted right sacrococcygeal sidebending
- sensitive or painful left sacrococcygeal sidebending
- restricted left sacrococcygeal sidebending.

If your score (one to seven checkmarks) is five or more, internal manipulation is recommended. If the score is three or less, the coccygeal problem is usually compensation for a distant mechanical disturbance (myofascial, visceral, or dura mater tension).

Manual cranial differential diagnosis

Local listening

Location of cranial restrictions by local listening is fairly easy. Analysis and differential diagnosis can be much more difficult.

Sutural restrictions

These attract your hand in a localized and precise manner. Usually, the palm of your hand undergoes rapid pronation or supination. The attraction is strong but not very deep.

A significant sutural restriction tends to restrict the neighboring dura mater. Usually, the coronal suture reflects restrictions of all the other cranial sutures. It is unusual for it to be free after significant skull trauma or dura mater injury.

Fractures

We often diagnose cranial fractures missed by x-ray examination. The palm is drawn in a more global way than the linear pulling typical of sutural restrictions, and there is usually also an axial rotation. The thenar or hypothenar eminence ends up over the fracture zone.

Cerebral tissue restrictions

There are a huge number of possible cerebral tissue lesions. Your hand is capable of detecting tissue which is either abnormally dense or loose as can occur with neoplasms, *but without being able to definitively diagnose the problem*. Your palm is drawn to this zone deep inside the skull, as if by a magnet, and gives the impression of being stuck. If you feel this type of pulling, refer the patient to a specialist.

We have found a dozen cerebral tumors in this way. Four of the patients had undergone examinations with negative results (including EEG and CT scan) within a few weeks before we saw them. The tumors were identified after we convinced the patient to have the imaging studies redone.

In epilepsy, the palm of your hand (usually the hypothenar eminence) is attracted deeply in the direction of the lateral part of the falx. Compared to the pull from a cyst or tumor, that from epilepsy starts out direct and precise, but becomes less so at the end.

The sensory system

Eyes

If the palm is drawn superficially and laterally toward the fronto-orbital region, there is often desynchronization of ocular movement, or asymmetrical tension of one or both eyes. This can mean obvious strabismus in which the eye is strongly drawn to one side, or covert strabismus in which the eyes appear well-balanced, but at the expense of strong compensatory muscle activity. Ocular muscle problems may reflect compensations for sutural or dura mater restrictions. This usually involves a cervical restriction on the same side, leading eventually to cervicobrachial neuralgia or spinal pain.

All ocular problems can be detected by local listening. In the case of muscular problems we have a specific "eyeball test."

EYEBALL TEST

Gently grasp the eyeball through the eyelid between the index finger and thumb and mobilize it in all three planes. Difficulty in mobilizing the eye in one direction indicates a muscular problem on the opposite side. This is often seen following fetal stress, which is associated with restriction of the coronal suture on the same side. Dura mater tension can restrict the eyeball because of extension of the dura on the optic nerve.

INHIBITION TEST

Suppose that you find a sutural or dura mater area which is fixed on the right side, together with a positive ipsilateral eyeball test. In the same listening position, you inhibit the ocular muscle tension by gently mobilizing the eye toward its restriction (indirect technique). Disappearance of the local listening proves the existence of an ocular muscle problem. Any remaining pull on listening indicates a dura mater, sutural, or intracranial problem which needs to be released.

We can also use the aggravation test, that is, increasing muscular tension of the eye and evaluating potential increase of local cranial listening. For example, suppose that on local listening you feel a pull toward the right eye, and during the eyeball test you feel a restriction when you attempt to move this eye laterally. Inhibition would then involve moving the right eye medially while your other hand does local listening. If the pull toward the right eye on listening were unclear, it would become clearer when you move this eye laterally.

VISUAL ZONES

When there are defects in the visual zones, we obtain positive posterolateral occipitoparietal listening which does not extend beyond the lambdoid sutures. The palm slides laterally backward, but is not very strongly drawn.

Ears

For problems in this area, the palm is drawn toward the petrous part of the temporal, anterior to location for the visual zones. For the ear itself, the palm slides laterally toward the ear. It exerts a slight supination for the right ear, and a pronation for the left ear. For the auditory zones, the palm slides slightly laterally behind the ear orifice. There is only slight listening, and the palm is directed more anterolaterally than it is for the visual zones. Problems of the auditory zones are often accompanied by ipsilateral cervical restriction, and the subject inclines the head to obtain the most effective position for hearing.

Visceral Manual Diagnosis

The spleen, left kidney, thorax, and neck organs are the visceral structures most often affected by severe trauma. We shall first discuss the left-sided distribution of the forces of collision.

Left visceral lesions

In our consultations, we are often surprised by the relative frequency and severity of visceral lesions on the left side, primarily following thoracoabdominal trauma. The forces of collision are typically concentrated on, for example, the left kidney, spleen, and left edge of the liver (left triangular ligament). These visceral injuries have local mechanical repercussions and affect general health.

Although visceral injuries can also occur on the right side, they are clearly more common on the left. We have a theory regarding this phenomenon. Our explanation is undoubtedly only one of many possibilities, but it is based on a logical use of anatomical data.

Distribution of the forces of collision

When upper and middle thoracic trauma occurs during a car accident, the forces of collision are absorbed by the skeleton and intrathoracic organs. Without the thoracic organs, the thoracic cage would have minimal resistance and break upon minor impact. The forces of collision follow the direction given by the organs and soft tissues of the thorax *(Fig. 5-43)*.

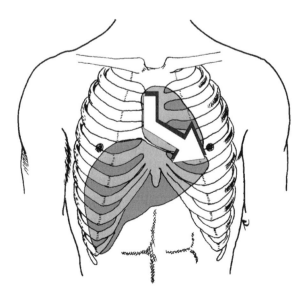

Fig. 5-43: Preferential orientation of the distribution of traumatic forces inside the thorax

The forces are also exerted upward, and are partially dissipated by the mobility of the cervical column. The cervicothoracic junction receives a large part of these upward forces of collision, which may account for the frequency with which post-traumatic lower cervical restrictions are accompanied by elongation of the cervicopleural attachments.

When the head is not supported by a headrest, the upper cervical vertebrae receive much of the force. Posteriorly, the shock waves are directed at the rigid spinal column, which reflects most of them anterolaterally. Next, the sternum and ribs send the shock waves to the central part of the thorax, where their only option is to follow the directions given by the anatomic conformation of the intrathoracic viscera.

HEART

Forces of collision concentrated in the thorax first affect the mediastinum, pericardium, and heart. The heart, surrounded by its large vessels, forms a mass which is denser than the lung, but it is still a hollow and elastic organ. It absorbs part of the shock waves and distributes the rest downward and to the left, as dictated by its orientation and major axis. Its elasticity may allow it to reflect and redirect the force of collision, like a rubber ball.

PERICARDIAL BASE

When we examine the zone of adherence of the pericardium to the diaphragm, we realize that its major axis is directed obliquely from the back to the front and from right to left. More specifically, the right edge is slightly oblique posteriorly and medially, while the left edge is strongly oblique from back to front and from right to left. The major axis of the base of the heart is tilted from the top to the bottom, from right to left, and from back to front. It is closer to the horizontal than to the vertical.

In conclusion, forces of collision are directed laterally to the left and not in an inferior direction, as one might assume. Research on the mediastinum by our friend and colleague Jean-Jacques Papassin (1991) confirms the preponderant role of this asymmetry.

DIAPHRAGM

The heart follows the movements of the diaphragm. During inhalation, it moves superiorly, posteriorly, and medially. As first noted by Testut, its mobility is greatest (~1 to 3cm) in the left lateral decubitus position.

During trauma, respiration temporarily ceases and the diaphragm may go into spasm. The diaphragm is higher on the left than on the right side. This diaphragmatic asymmetry is another factor in the left-sided distribution of the forces of collision during trauma. The diaphragm constitutes a hard, smooth plane which propagates the forces of collision toward its most sloping sections.

SPLEEN AND LEFT KIDNEY

Because they are situated below and to the left of the heart and diaphragm, it is understandable that these organs receive a large part of the forces of collision:

- the spleen, which is a fragile organ, may crack or break from the shock
- the kidney, which is denser, more solid and resistant, may crack (leading to hematuria) or undergo compression and great stretching of the posterior attach-

ments. This stretching has pathological consequences on the diaphragm and the esophageal/cardiac/gastric junction. When it is unable to return a large part of the forces of collision, the kidney loses its natural position and undergoes ptosis.

We will return later to the left kidney and spleen, which are so often affected by trauma. Before then, we will consider other visceral tissues of the thorax and neck.

Thorax

The thorax contains approximately 150 joints. Simultaneous small movements at many joints allow the entire structure to move and change shape, making the thorax highly adaptable. A tissue restriction following trauma is usually asymptomatic during a period of latency. If the thorax is relatively free mechanically before the trauma, signs of mechanical decompensation will not become evident for a long time.

The thorax is a cavity with constant subatmospheric pressure, and its walls and organs are highly interdependent. Forces of trauma are usually concentrated at the superior thoracic outlet. Whereas the cervical segment is very mobile, the thoracic segment is relatively rigid. The cervicothoracic junction is, therefore, an area of conflicting mechanical influences. During whiplash or other trauma, the forces of collision tend to converge toward this transitional zone and overload it with mechanical stress. Many pericardial and pleural structures have their insertions in this area. Certain factors, such as a seat belt, increase the concentration of forces on the superior thoracic outlet.

Crossed mediastinal test

Your first step is to locate the traumatic injury to the thoracic tissues, which will clarify their loss of elasticity and site of restriction. Position yourself on the patient's right side, and place the heel of your left hand on the second right intercostal space, level with the sternum, with the fingers directed along the longitudinal axis of the heart. Place your right hand over your left hand, to give symmetrical support *(Fig. 5-44)*.

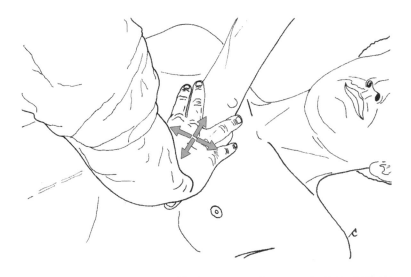

Fig. 5-44: Crossed mediastinal test

"Stack" the tissues by exerting progressive inward pressure with your hands, visualizing and feeling the different tissue layers. When you feel the heart beating under your hands, you have reached the ideal depth for this test. By maintaining tissue stacking at a proper depth, you induce movement by first pushing the cardiac mass along its longitudinal axis:

- inferiorly and to the left
- superiorly and to the right.

Then, perpendicular to this axis:

- inferiorly and to the right
- superiorly and to the left.

Testing in these four directions enables you to evaluate, two by two, the four major tissue sectors.

- The slight stretching that you cause enables you to locate the restricted side. You stretch the right-side structures by pushing to the left, and vice versa.
- A push inferiorly tests the pericardial suspensory systems and to a lesser extent the superior pleural attachments and visceral sheath of the neck.
- A push superiorly gives information on the elasticity of the phrenopericardial ligaments and diaphragm muscle, and related visceral abdominal restrictions (e.g., of the hepatic ligaments, spleen, stomach, kidneys).

This test provides a global approach to visceral restrictions of the thorax. It allows quick diagnosis of the most significant restrictions, and location of the zone most affected by the trauma.

Tests of the pleural dome

Because of its anatomical complexity, mechanical injury to the pleural dome may produce a variety of symptoms. Structures found at the pleural dome include the following *(Fig. 5-45)*:

- subclavian artery, and its collateral branches at this level (vertebral, internal thoracic, and inferior thyroid artery)
- lower roots of the brachial plexus
- inferior cervical ganglion and the anastomatic subclavian loop (also known as Vieussens' ansa)
- phrenic nerve.

Stimulation or irritation of any of these elements may cause symptoms at distant sites of the body.

BILATERAL TEST OF THE PLEURAL DOME

This rapid test enables you to feel restrictions of the suspensory tissues. Stand behind the seated patient, with the occiput and superior thoracic region against you. Place your index fingers just behind the medial ends of the clavicles, with your fingertips on the scalene (Lisfranc's) tubercles of the first ribs, where the anterior scalenes insert.

Induce cervicothoracic tension centered on C7-T1 until you feel the anterolateral muscles of the neck begin to relax. Continue with the tips of your index fingers inside

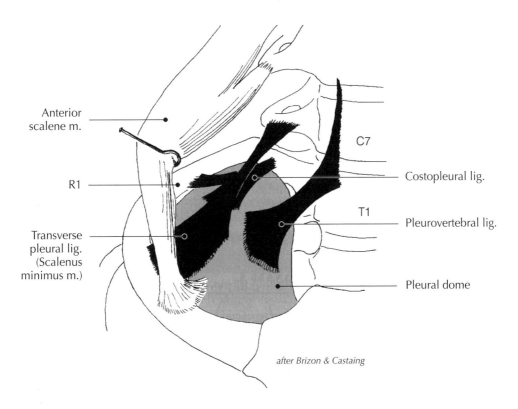

Fig. 5-45: Suspensory apparatus of the pleural dome

(medial and inferior to) the scalene tubercles, pressing to make sure that you are well inside the internal circumference of the first rib.

Place your middle finger above your index to make your support as flexible as possible. Alternately push on the lower part of each pleural dome, posteromedially, to evaluate the elasticity of each suspensory apparatus. Restriction of the suspensory ligaments is characterized by a distinct feeling that the pleural dome refuses to be compressed.

SPECIFIC TEST OF THE PLEURAL DOME

After diagnosing the side with the restriction, you should clarify the ligament involved. There are three principal ligaments:

- *transverse pleural ligament:* oblique inferiorly and laterally, it extends from the transverse process of C7 to the lateral aspect of the pleural dome and the first rib. In many people, this structure contains muscle fibers and is known as the scalenus minimus muscle.
- *pleurovertebral ligament:* almost vertical, slightly oblique inferiorly and laterally. It extends from the prevertebral aponeurosis near the vertebral body of C7 and part of C6 and T1, to the medial aspect of the pleural dome.
- *costopleural ligament:* almost horizontal in its superior part and then slightly oblique anteriorly, laterally, and inferiorly, it extends from the neck of the first rib to the posterior lateral aspect of the pleural dome.

To evaluate the elasticity of each specific ligament, we create a fixed point on the pleural dome and test it by exerting slight traction from the cervicothoracic column.

Stand behind the seated patient. To test the right pleural dome, use your left hand and forearm to slightly right sidebend the cervical column, trying to focus the movement on the C7/T1 region. This permits the muscular masses of the subclavicular region to relax.

With your middle finger over the tip of the right index finger as in the bilateral test, delicately penetrate the tissues inside the scalene tubercle and create a fixed point by maintaining the pleural dome inferiorly, posteriorly, and inward. You can then evaluate each ligament by creating a slight movement of the cervical column, as follows *(Fig. 5-46)*:

- pure left sidebending, to test the transverse pleural ligament
- left sidebending and right rotation, to test the costopleural ligament
- left sidebending and left rotation, to test the pleurovertebral ligament.

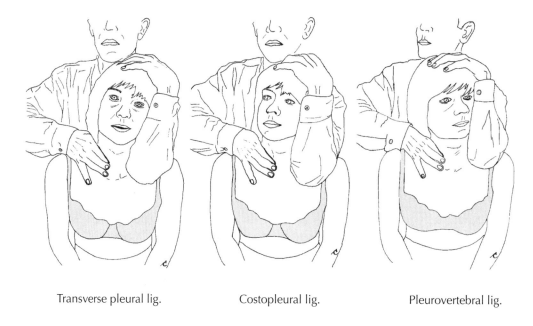

Transverse pleural lig.   Costopleural lig.   Pleurovertebral lig.

Fig. 5-46: Specific tests of the suspensory ligaments of the pleural dome

You should feel the elasticity of each ligament during this movement. There is a latent period between cervicothoracic stress and reaction to it on the pleural dome.

In the case of ligamentous restriction, elasticity is minimal or absent, and the cervical movement immediately places the ligament under tension. As a result, the pleural dome "ejects" the index finger which formed the fixed point. Our students have often been surprised to note that a single ligament may be restricted while the other two have normal elasticity.

Visceral sheath of the neck

All the visceral, vascular, and nervous elements of the neck are united and isolated by a fibrous sheath referred to as the *visceral sheath of the neck*. This fascial system maintains the fragile anterior elements of the neck:

- vascular, nervous: carotid arteries, jugular veins, vagus nerves
- digestive: pharynx, upper esophagus
- respiratory: larynx, trachea
- endocrine: thyroid, parathyroid.

In addition to maintaining and compartmentalizing these elements, this fascial system permits the cervical viscera to slide with and in front of the cervical column. In fact, within the fibrous sheath there is a space with retropharyngeal and retroesophageal gliding that acts as a true visceral joint.

Don't assume that these movements are small! The distance from the hyoid bone to the sternum can double with cervical extension. The viscera of the neck must be able to glide in front of the cervical vertebrae in order to adjust to such variations in length.

The fibrous sheath is secured:

- superiorly, by the pharyngobasilar fascia under the basilar part of the occipital, the apex of the petrous portion of the temporals, and the lower part of the posterior sphenoid *(Fig. 5-47)*. Note that this attachment is at the point of intersection of four bones of the base of the cranium. (These superior insertions cross over the sphenobasilar symphysis, which explains the disastrous consequences on the PRM of a visceral restriction of the neck.)
- posteriorly, to the top of the cervical column via the prevertebral lamina of cervical fascia, which also attaches it to the prevertebral aponeurosis *(Fig. 5-48)*.
- inferiorly, to the pericardial system via the thyropericardial lamina, an extension of which is weakened near the base of the visceral sheath.

During major cervical trauma (vertebral fracture, sprain, dislocation, whiplash), the visceral sheath of the neck may be affected in two ways:

- elongation of visceral attachments during the cervical extension phase, which may cause tears or micro-tears of the securing fibers. Secondary wound phenomena may lead to sclerosis and tissue fibrosis, and resulting loss of elasticity limits movements of the visceral sheath.
- edema or hematoma behind the visceral sheath. The retained fluid gradually spreads through the virtual gliding spaces, causing sticking, loss of motion, and localized restriction of the visceral sheath.

To emphasize the significance of these phenomena, we tell our students that visceral restrictions of the neck play the same role in cervical mechanics as that played by visceral abdominal restrictions in abdominal/lumbar mechanics!

Because of the great mobility of the cervical column and its intimate links with the visceral sheath of the neck, any interference with normal movement of neck viscera or vessels will restrict cervical mechanics over the short or long term. Recurrent cervical restrictions observed in the absence of significant joint dysfunction illustrate this phenomenon.

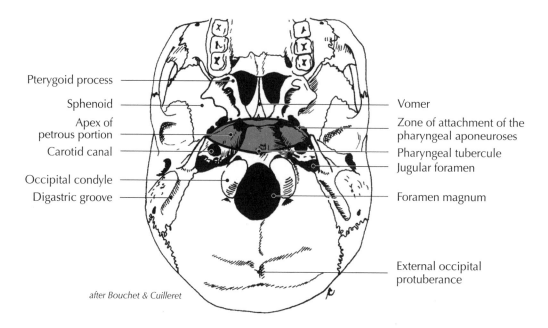

after Bouchet & Cuilleret

Fig. 5-47: Superior attachments of the visceral sheath of the neck by the pharyngeal aponeuroses

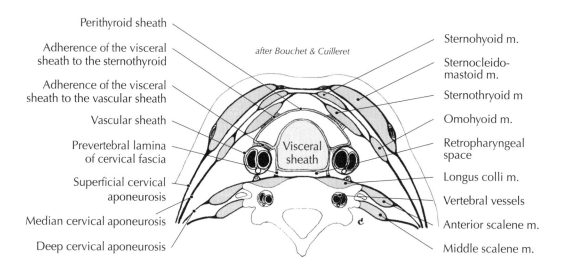

after Bouchet & Cuilleret

Fig. 5-48: Schematic section of C6

Three-fingered test of the visceral sheath

Stand or sit at the head of the supine patient. Approach the visceral sheath of the neck at the level of the retropharyngeal and retroesophageal gliding spaces, immediately anterior to the transverse processes. The approach should be symmetrical on both sides to avoid misinterpretation. Place the index finger on the inferior part of the neck, immediately above the clavicle, the middle finger on the middle section, and the ring finger on the superior part, immediately behind the most posterolateral point ("gonion") on the external angle of the mandible *(Fig. 5-49)*.

Approach the tissues transversely, and locate the plane of gliding to make sure that your support is perfectly symmetrical. Place the little fingers on the horizontal ramus of the mandible to limit rotation of the head during the mobility test. Join your thumbs in a fulcrum in front of the throat to stabilize your hands and make the test more reliable.

Perform gliding movements to the right and left, and also upward and downward to evaluate the retropharyngeal articulation.

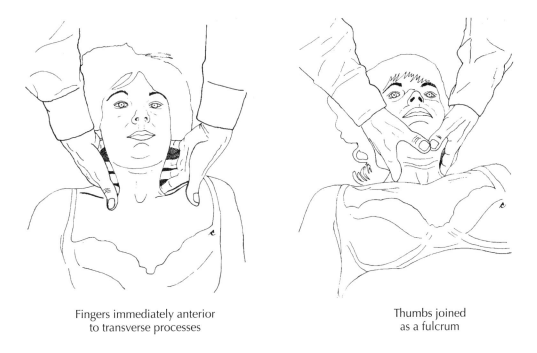

Fingers immediately anterior
to transverse processes

Thumbs joined
as a fulcrum

Fig. 5-49: Three-finger test of the visceral sheath of the neck

The visceral sheath of the neck is usually mobile symmetrically relative to the median axis. It should be mobile upward and downward.

Try to "unstick" the visceral sheath from the cervical column to evaluate the elasticity of the prevertebral laminae of the cervical fascia. It is usually possible to draw the sheath forward a short distance. In the event that the prevertebral laminae are restricted (typically unilaterally), you will note an asymmetry of movement. Loss of elasticity (restriction) on one side tends to make the visceral sheath rotate to that side.

Left kidney

The left kidney must always be considered when treating trauma victims. Manipulation of this organ, its attachments, and gliding surfaces yields excellent results on its restrictions and associated loss of energy. We will focus here on a posterior approach to this organ, since we have described an anterior approach in earlier books

(Barral and Mercier, 1988 and Barral, 1989), and because posterior restrictions are more pathogenic from a mechanical and energetic point of view. Interestingly, a posterior restriction of the left kidney almost always leads to restriction of the left first rib and C7, indicating its effect on the myofascial system.

Posterior approach

Above

The left kidney is closer to the thoracic cavity than is the right kidney. The upper two thirds of its posterior surface are in contact with the thoracics, as opposed to only the upper half of the right kidney *(Fig. 5-50)*.

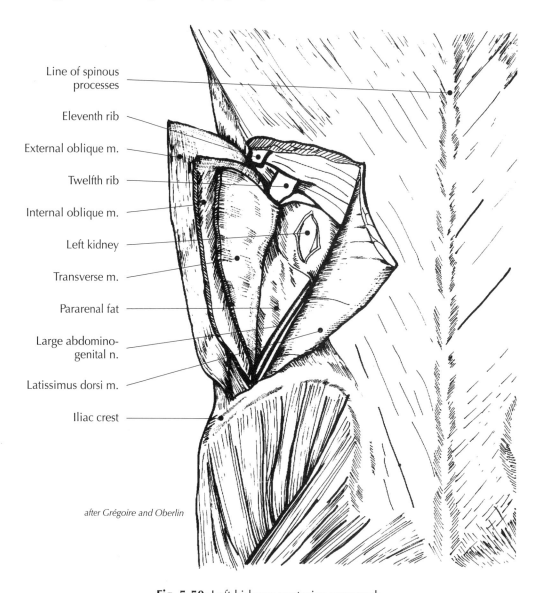

Line of spinous processes

Eleventh rib

External oblique m.

Twelfth rib

Internal oblique m.

Left kidney

Transverse m.

Pararenal fat

Large abdomino-genital n.

Latissimus dorsi m.

Iliac crest

after Grégoire and Oberlin

Fig. 5-50: Left kidney: posterior approach

The diaphragmatic fibers facing the posterior surface of the left kidney form a very thin lamina, which inserts on the internal diaphragmatic arch and the lateral part of the quadratus lumborum muscle. The diaphragmatic septum has a costodiaphragmatic hiatus in the form of a triangle whose lower base corresponds to the arch of the quadratus lumborum and to the twelfth rib.

At this level, the posterior surface of the kidney is in direct contact with the inferior pleural cul de sac, and its lower third is supported by the quadratus lumborum. The twelfth intercostal, iliohypogastric, and ilioinguinal nerves are located within the cellular-adipose mass between the aponeurosis of the quadratus lumborum and the postrenal fascia. This accounts for the genital pain sometimes associated with trauma to the kidney and ureters.

BELOW

The kidney extends beyond the lateral border of the quadratus lumborum, and has close links with the transversus abdominis. There are two weak points in this area, as described below.

Grynfelt's triangle is a triangular space bounded superiorly by the twelfth rib and the inferior posterior serratus muscle, anteriorly by the internal oblique, posteriorly by the quadratus lumborum, and medially by the paravertebral musculature *(Fig. 5-51)*. Posterior manipulation of the kidney is done through this space.

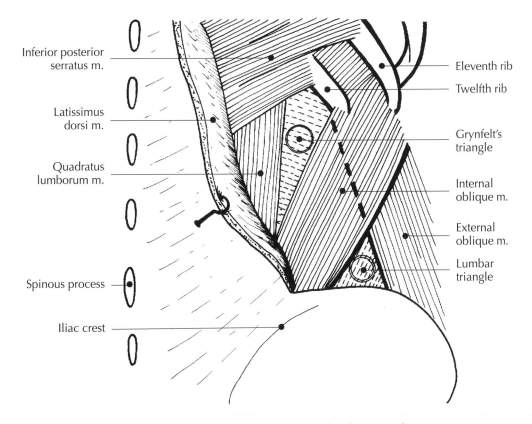

Fig. 5-51: Grynfelt's triangle and the lumbar triangle

The lumbar triangle is bounded above by the crossing over of the latissimus dorsi and the external obliques, inferiorly by the iliac crest, anteriorly and laterally by the external obliques, and posteriorly and laterally by the latissimus dorsi and paravertebrals.

Anterior approach

In anterior view the left kidney relates superiorly to the tail of the pancreas, superiorly and laterally to the spleen (which partially covers it), and at its midpoint to the terminal portion of the transverse colon (primarily to its mesocolon) and the initial portion of the descending colon. The left kidney has more connections with the transverse and descending colon than the right kidney has with the transverse and ascending colons. It relates to the posterior surface of the stomach via the posterior parietal peritoneum *(Figs. 5-52 & 5-53)*. The transverse mesocolon attaches to the anterior portion of the left kidney, placing it both above and below the mesocolon.

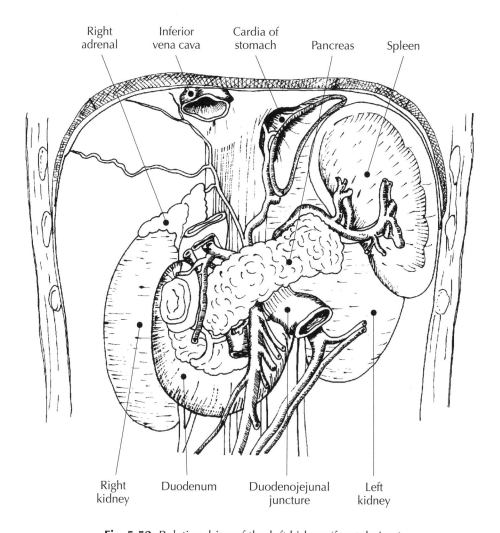

Fig. 5-52: Relationships of the left kidney (frontal view)

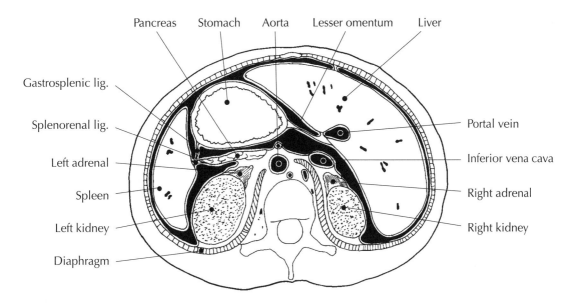

Pancreas   Stomach   Aorta   Lesser omentum   Liver

Gastrosplenic lig.

Splenorenal lig.

Left adrenal

Spleen

Left kidney

Diaphragm

Portal vein

Inferior vena cava

Right adrenal

Right kidney

Fig. 5-53: Relationships of the left kidney (horizontal view)

Medially, the left kidney is close to the transverse processes, in particular those of L1. This vertebra is frequently fractured from falls on the buttocks, heels, or back, and in automobile accidents. The left kidney is affected by shock waves concentrated at L1, and must be mobilized after L1 fractures. Cases of lower back pain following an L1 fracture are often related to renal problems.

The upper pole of the left kidney is hidden under the diaphragm, and the adrenal gland is medial to the most superior point. In cases of renal ptosis, the adrenal gland does not follow the kidney; it always remains in its place. The upper pole is at the level of rib 11 and is closely related to the pleura. The lower pole is at the level of the upper edge of the transverse process of L3, ~5cm from the iliac crest.

Consequences of these relationships

Grynfelt's triangle is generally the most direct and best route for posterior manipulation of the left kidney. The left kidney has important connections with the last two ribs, the pleura, and the first rib (via the pleura). Because of its relationship with the transverse colon and mesocolon, spleen, pancreas, and stomach, therapeutic manipulation of the left kidney should always include mobilization and release of these organs.

Symptoms and clinical signs of left kidney restrictions

Lower back pain occurs at the vertebral and sacroiliac level, and radiates toward the left flank. On palpation, there is a clear difference between the two Grynfelt's triangles: on the side of the restricted kidney, it is more easily felt, and more difficult to press in with the thumb or fingers.

Abdominal pain often follows the path of the twelfth intercostal nerve. There may be a deep sensation of *heaviness in the abdomen* that radiates toward the surface, erroneously attributed to a functional colon problem. In general, lower back pain and sensation of abdominal heaviness are more frequent in the early morning and late evening hours.

The patient experiences *thigh pain* or paresthesia in the area innervated by the lateral femoral cutaneous nerve (primarily the lateral surface of the thigh).

Left renal restriction often leads to lower left *cervical pain* or restriction through the myofascial chains. We learned to focus on the kidney after repeated failures with local cervical manipulation in these patients. This and similar experiences taught us that true vertebral restriction is bilateral. A unilateral "vertebral" restriction almost always reflects compensation for a problem elsewhere.

Left first rib restriction is often observed following tissue trauma involving the left kidney and spleen, usually as a result of disequilibrium of an underlying ipsilateral ligamentous/fascial chain. Do not start with local manipulation; this is usually ineffective and may even cause painful and lasting cervicobrachial neuralgia.

Left shoulder pain ranges from simple discomfort to scapulohumeral periarthritis. These symptoms are also found in splenic restrictions.

Blood pressure may vary during the day. Most commonly, there is cyclic hypotension in the late morning and afternoon.

Urogenital problems range from genital pain (related to the iliohypogastric, ilioinguinal, or genitofemoral nerve) to urinary infection and sexual dysfunction.

Loss of energy can be profound. The patient can carry out essential activities, but is not truly active or creative.

Tests of kidney mobility

There are two useful tests using a posterior approach to the left kidney.

SUPINE POSITION

The patient is supine, arms resting on the chest, left leg bent. Stand facing the left flank and place the lateral edge of your right index finger between the iliac crest and the left twelfth rib (around the transverse process L3), and your thumb on the corresponding lateral part. Your elbow is bent, and pressed against your chest. Your thumb is pressing on the latissimus dorsi and the posterolateral part of the descending colon. Check the mobility via the index finger in Grynfelt's triangle, moving it cephalad, medially, and anteriorly.

When there is a renal restriction, it may be difficult to place the index finger between the iliac crest and rib 12. The area seems overly firm and only slightly compressible, and the patient feels pain or discomfort. In this case, advance your finger more slowly, reduce the pressure, and repeat the test several times in a rhythmic manner until you have a good sense of the restriction.

Next, place the palm of your left hand on the abdomen, at the level of the duodenojejunal junction, and direct it posteriorly, slightly medially, and superiorly. The palm ends up on the anterior part of the inferior pole of the left kidney.

Using both hands, mobilize the kidney anteriorly, medially, and superiorly *(Fig. 5-54)*. With a restriction, anterior movement is difficult. You can use respiration to feel the kidney fall during inhalation and rise during exhalation.

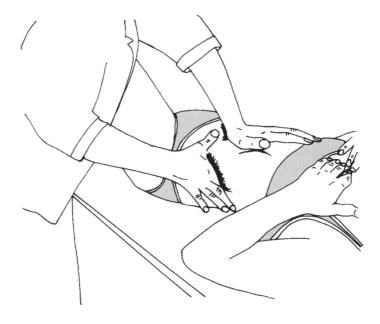

Fig. 5-54: Mobility test of left kidney: supine position

Right lateral decubitus position

In front of the patient

The patient lies on the right side, right leg extended, left leg bent, and head resting on a cushion or on the flexed right forearm. Standing in front of the patient, place your right thumb in Grynfelt's triangle, your palm resting on the paravertebral mass and the iliac crest. Your left palm exerts active counter-support on the lateral part of the left costochondral joints *(Fig. 5-55)*.

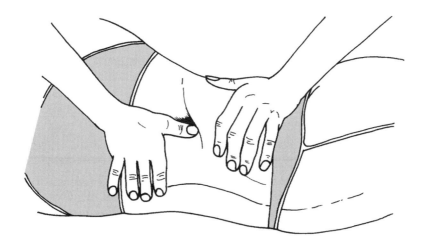

Fig. 5-55: Mobility test of left kidney:
right lateral decubitus position from in front of patient

Push your right thumb anteriorly, medially, and superiorly, while mobilizing the left rib cage to increase penetration of your thumb in Grynfelt's triangle. A renal restriction is indicated if Grynfelt's triangle is firm and resists compression by your thumb. You can ask the patient to breathe while you evaluate myofascial tension in the area.

Behind the patient

The patient is in the same position, but you stand behind her. If you position yourself relatively near the head, your left thumb is in Grynfelt's triangle and the rest of your hand is on the right side of the back. Your right hand, placed on the left lateral abdomen, pushes posteriorly and superiorly to mobilize the kidney for evaluation *(Fig. 5-56)*.

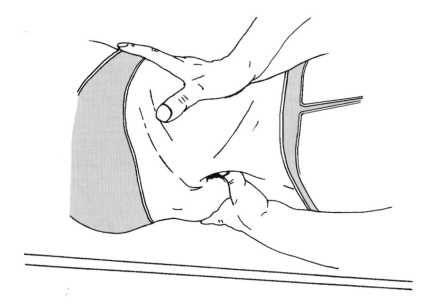

Fig. 5-56: Mobility test of left kidney: right lateral decubitus position from behind patient

Alternatively, you can position yourself closer to the feet, with your right thumb against Grynfelt's triangle, the rest of your right hand pressed against the latissimus dorsi and paravertebral mass, and your elbow against your right hip. Your left hand pushes the left rib cage posteriorly and laterally, while your right thumb pushes anteriorly, medially, and superiorly on Grynfelt's triangle *(Fig. 5-57)*.

LISTENING TEST

In the positions described above, when your thumbs have achieved maximum penetration, slightly relax the pressure and allow them to follow the direction of listening. As usual, listening permits you to be more specific in identifying areas of restriction.

Novice practitioners tend to press too hard on any area which is difficult to feel. This is counterproductive because if you trigger pain, the muscles in the affected area (in this case, the iliocostal region) will contract to guard the area from further harm, so that listening is even more difficult.

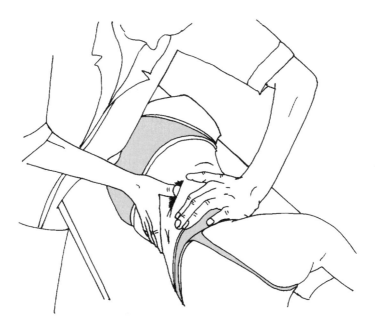

Fig. 5-57: Mobility test of left kidney: right lateral decubitus position from behind patient (2nd method)

These techniques frequently cause a slight feeling of discomfort, especially if the kidney is restricted, *but never real pain.* In the event of pain, you should immediately relax the pressure of your thumb and change direction. Repeat this as many times as necessary to feel clearly without causing pain.

Osteoarticular relationships

Osteoarticular restrictions relating to the left kidney are located primarily at the level of T7-T11, L1, R1, R11, R12, and the left sacroiliac. You should first manipulate the left kidney, and only then treat remaining osteoarticular restrictions.

Spleen

This organ is very difficult to grasp from an osteopathic or physiological point of view. Only after fifteen years of work have we become slightly familiar with it. We will describe its attachments and relationships with neighboring structures, all of which are affected by manipulation of the spleen.

Anatomy of the spleen

The average spleen is 13cm long, 5cm wide, and weighs 150-200g. Testut (1896) considered it the softest and least resistant of all the glandular organs. Its low resistance accounts in part for its frequent injury during trauma. Its position is maintained by peritoneal folds, which are omental rather than ligamentous.

SPLENIC COMPARTMENT

The conceptual compartment of the spleen *(Fig. 5-58)* is bordered:

- superiorly, by a horizontal plane passing through rib 5
- inferiorly, by a horizontal plane at the inferior edge of the thorax
- laterally, by a plane tangent to the lateral wall of the thorax
- medially, by a vertical plane passing anterior to the nipple
- posteriorly, by the left lateral surface of the thoracic spine.

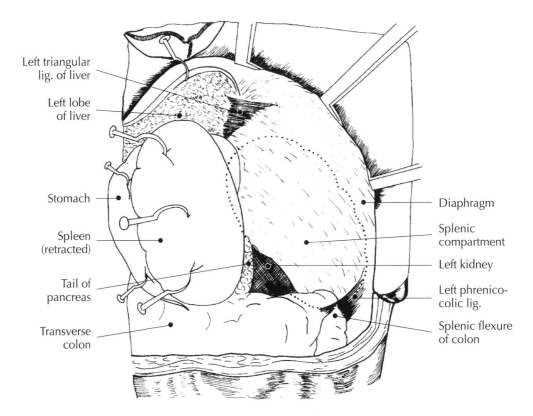

Fig. 5-58: Splenic compartment

RELATIONSHIPS

The lateral or phrenico-costal surface connects to the diaphragm and pleural cavity. It faces the left ribs 9, 10, and 11. The anteromedial or gastric surface relates to the posterior surface and greater curvature of the stomach. The posteromedial or renal surface presents a concave surface adapted to the anterior surfaces (lateral third of the upper half) of the left kidney and left adrenal. The left kidney and the spleen are separated only by a double peritoneal fold, and renal-splenic restrictions are common following infection or trauma. The basal surface is small and easily confused with the gastric surface. It rests upon the tail of the pancreas posteriorly, and the splenic flexure of the colon anteriorly.

SUPERIOR AND INFERIOR POLES

Some of the surfaces of the spleen are not relevant to testing or treatment. Our concern is mainly with the superior and inferior poles, through which we can sometimes exert an effect.

The *superior pole* is medial, and located very close (1-2cm) to T10. During trauma, the spleen may be projected against the spinal column and rupture.

The *inferior pole* is lateral, and lodged in a virtual "cradle" formed by the superior surface of the left phrenicocolic ligament. This ligament is the most important support of the spleen, and its manipulation is essential in treating splenic restrictions.

Attachments of the spleen

The peritoneum completely surrounds the spleen. One can affect the spleen via the omentum, splenic ligaments, and organs attached to them. Certain structures do not normally function as attachments, but can form restrictions with the spleen in the aftermath of trauma.

The *gastrosplenic ligament* extends from the greater curvature of the stomach to the hilum of the spleen, and is 3-4cm in length.

The *splenorenal ligament* contains the vascular pedicle of the spleen and the tail of the pancreas, and is also known as the pancreaticosplenic ligament. It is 2-3cm long and extends from the hilum of the spleen to the parietal peritoneum. It contacts the anterior surface of the left kidney, adrenal gland, and neighboring part of the diaphragm.

The *phrenicosplenic ligament*, when present, links the pancreas and spleen to the diaphragm.

The *splenocolic ligament* is a small omental fold running from the inferior edge of the spleen to the transverse colon, very close to its splenic flexure.

SPLENIC FLEXURE OF THE TRANSVERSE COLON

This flexure is situated deeply between the lateral edge of the left kidney and the abdominal wall, in the renal parietal sinus. Its manipulation permits release of splenic restrictions.

The splenic flexure has a sharper angle than the hepatic flexure, and is more superior and posterior. It has three major layers of attachment. The superficial attachment is the left phrenicocolic ligament. The middle layer is composed of the gastrosplenic and (when present) pancreaticosplenic ligaments. The deep layer is the left edge of Toldt's fascia, which connects the posterior colon to the posterior parietal peritoneum.

In contrast to the right side, the left side of the transverse colon is linked to the posterior parietal peritoneum by a long mesocolon, which gives a greater degree of mobility. The transverse colon joins the lumbar wall laterally near the left kidney.

LEFT PHRENICOCOLIC LIGAMENT

This is the most important attachment of the descending colon and the spleen. It extends from the posterior parietal peritoneum and the diaphragm to the splenic flexure of the colon. The inferior pole of the spleen sits in the hollow of its superior surface, and was referred to as the "cradle of the spleen" by early anatomists. This ligament sends extensions to all the organs surrounding the spleen, and mobilizing it also affects the stomach, transverse and descending colon, left kidney, and pancreas *(Fig. 5-59)*.

Conclusions

The spleen is dependent upon the following structures:

- transverse colon, through the lateral edge of its mesocolon
- splenic flexure of colon, through the left phrenicocolic ligament

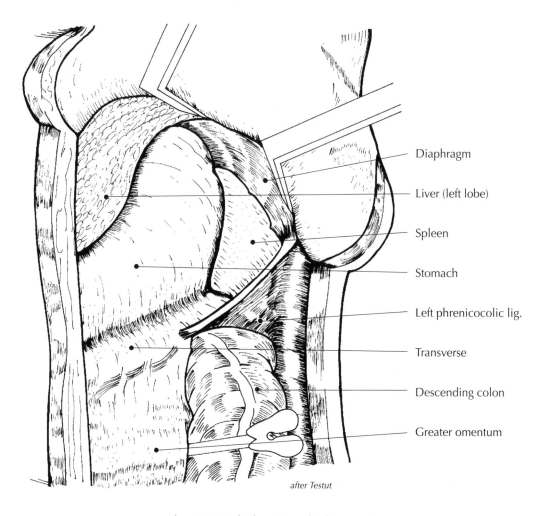

after Testut

Fig. 5-59: Left phrenicocolic ligament

- tail of the pancreas, through the deep middle layer of the left phrenicocolic ligament
- left kidney, through the deep layer of the left phrenicocolic ligament
- liver, through the left triangular ligament
- diaphragm, through the superficial layer of the left phrenicocolic ligament
- stomach, through the gastrosplenic ligament and middle layer of the left phrenicocolic ligament
- lumbar column, through the left crus of the diaphragm
- left ribs 5, 9, and 10
- T8 and T9, which correspond on a segmental level to the spleen and pancreas.

Position of the spleen is maintained by diaphragmatic attraction due to negative intrathoracic pressure, by the aspiration force of the blood flow, and by the turgor effect of neighboring hollow organs.

The spleen is most effectively manipulated through the:

- left phrenicocolic ligament
- left kidney
- splenic flexure of the colon
- transverse mesocolon
- stomach
- left ribs 8, 9, and 10
- T8-9.

Signs and symptoms of splenic restriction

Splenic restriction often occurs after an automobile accident or direct fall on the back. Clinical signs may take months or even years to appear, so that the patient does not associate them with the trauma. Principal signs include the following.

Abdominal discomfort. The patient feels deep discomfort in the area of the left hypochondrium which is difficult to localize with precision. The discomfort is easy to confuse with a renal problem or mechanical rib problem.

A *stitch in the side* involving the left side of the diaphragm while walking or running.

Left lower cervical pain with intertransverse restrictions of C4-C5-C6 often occurs after significant trauma of the spleen and neighboring structures.

Asthenia. The patient feels progressively more fatigued, wakes up tired, and finds all activity difficult. Since biological signs are nonexistent at first, the fatigue is often attributed to overwork or depression. The patient may feel insecure and abandoned, since the fatigue is real but doctors cannot account for it.

Splenic restrictions cause an *iron deficiency*, accompanied by hair loss, pallor and hypotonia, which may take months to occur. This can be treated by manipulating T9-10, their ribs, and the elements of the splenic compartment. When you see fatigue and iron deficiency with a history of trauma in children or adolescents, think of splenic dysfunction.

Lowered immune defenses. Patients with splenic restriction often suffer from ENT infections and chronic sore throats.

Micronodes. Small nodes shaped like a kernel of corn or a pea are often found at the cervical, subclavicular, axillary, and inguinal areas. They are less numerous than in infectious mononucleosis and are not accompanied by significant fever.

Hypotension and asymmetrical pressure. Systolic pressure can be around 10cm H_2O below normal in an adult. Also, pressure can be 10-20cm H_2O lower on the left than on the right side.

Muscular/ligamentous problems. The patient suffers repeated sprains, muscle pulls, and capsular/synovial inflammations.

Left scapulohumeral pain. This ranges from simple discomfort to periarthritis. The pain worsens with activity.

Left first rib restriction occurs frequently and is often secondary to abnormal tension of the fascial chains coming from the spleen and left kidney, or other ipsilateral mechanical disturbance located below.

Low-grade fever ranges near 37.5°C, particularly in the late afternoon or evening. Send these patients for complete medical evaluation.

Diagnosis of splenic restriction

The spleen is not easily found. This deeply situated and compressible organ is almost impossible to distinguish from neighboring organs such as left kidney, diaphragm, stomach, or cardiac base.

A spleen which is easily palpable is pathological and requires a careful workup. We have seen approximately 20 such patients, and most were unfortunately suffering from Hodgkin's disease or other types of lymphoma.

Splenic restriction may result from trauma such as an automobile accident or direct fall on the back or side, possibly a long time before the appearance of symptoms. Common signs (most were described above) include sensation of discomfort in the left hypochondrium, "stitch" in the diaphragm during activity, asthenia, iron deficiency, micronodes, depressed immune function, hypotension and asymmetrical blood pressure, low-grade fever, muscular/ligamentous problems, shoulder pain, and problems related to the left thoracic inlet.

Palpation and mobility tests for the spleen

We cannot really test mobility of the spleen itself. Splenic restriction is revealed by palpation of neighboring structures, associated with tests of mobility of the stomach, transverse colon, splenic flexure, left kidney, lower ribs, T11-12, and L1-2.

GASTROPHRENIC LIGAMENT TEST

This ligament links the greater curvature of the stomach to the diaphragm. Its posterior section sends several fibers to the splenic compartment, and these may become restricted.

The patient is seated, hands resting on the thighs. Standing behind the patient, use your left hand to push the left twelfth ribs anteromedially, so as to relax the gastrophrenic attachments.

Place the thumb or fingers of your right hand on the left edge of the rectus abdominis and press upward, backward, and slightly inward. Then lightly push the greater curvature of the stomach inferomedially *(Fig. 5-60)*. You can increase flexion of the trunk by adding slight rightward rotation and thereby facilitate your approach to the left posterolateral part of the gastrophrenic ligament.

If there is a restriction of this part of the ligament, you will feel an area which is more stretched, and experience some difficulty in pushing the stomach inferiorly and medially. A positive test does not prove splenic restriction, but is a strong indicator.

TRANSVERSE MESOCOLON TEST

This structure has important extensions toward the spleen, stomach, pancreas, splenic flexure, and posterior parietal peritoneum *(Fig. 5-61)*. There are two positions for testing the transverse mesocolon.

Supine position

The patient is supine, arms at the sides, legs bent. Standing or sitting behind the head, position your thumbs at the level of the tenth and eleventh costochondral joints, near the splenic and hepatic flexures *(Fig. 5-62)*. With your hands flattened, press your thumbs against the last ribs, in a posterior, medial, and inferior direction, and evaluate

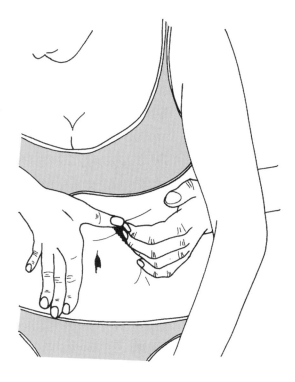

Fig. 5-60: Gastrophrenic ligament test

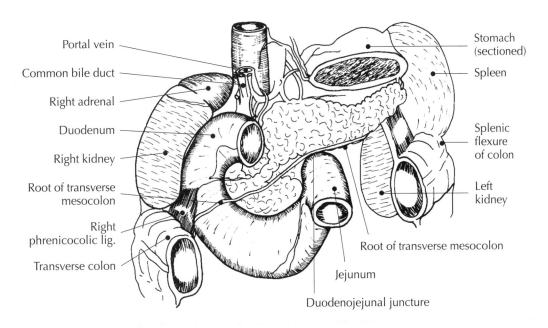

Fig. 5-61: Relationships of the transverse mesocolon

differences in tissue resistance to mobilization. During mobilization, your thumbs should remain on the transverse colon, near the flexures. The splenic flexure is higher and more posterior than the hepatic flexure. A restriction of the transverse mesocolon is revealed by resistance to stretching, and limited mobilization.

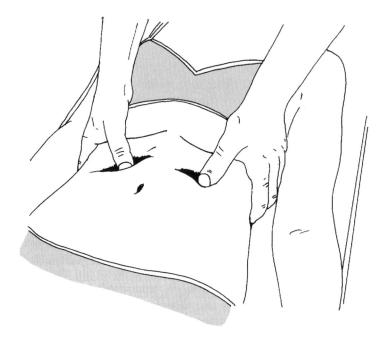

Fig. 5-62: Transverse mesocolon test (supine)

Seated position

The patient is seated, hands resting on the thighs, torso bent forward. Standing behind the patient, press your hands against the lateral surface of the last ribs with your two thumbs on the medial parts of the splenic and hepatic flexures of the colon, and push in a posterior, medial, inferior direction as above *(Fig. 5-63)*. The restriction is located in the area of least mobility.

Add sidebending and rotation of the flexed thorax to more easily explore the different portions of the transverse mesocolon. A rotation to the right permits evaluation of the left phrenicocolic portion, while rotation to the left improves contact with the gastrophrenic portion.

These two tests may be performed with listening techniques. During the mobilizations as above, let your hands be drawn in the direction of listening to locate the area of restriction.

LEFT PHRENICOCOLIC LIGAMENT TEST

Seated position

Stand behind the seated patient, with your right knee on the table. Place your left hand against the left rib cage and the fingers of your right hand subcostally, at the level

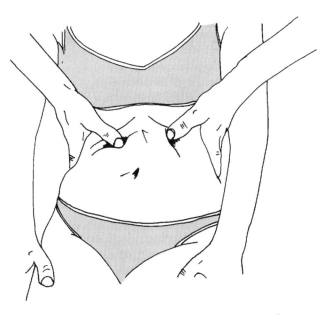

Fig. 5-63: Transverse mesocolon test (seated)

of the ninth through eleventh costochondral joints. Draw the rib cage medially, inferiorly, and anteriorly to relax the abdominals and permit better penetration of the right hand in the direction of the splenic flexure *(Fig. 5-64)*.

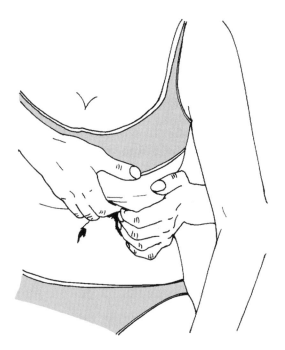

Fig. 5-64: Left phrenicocolic ligament test (seated)

With your right fingers, exert pressure on the different fibers of the left phrenico-colic ligament. Try to compare the fibers which traverse the mesocolon, those running in the direction of the diaphragm and stomach, and the more lateral and posterior fibers going toward the spleen. With practice, you can evaluate the thickness and distensibility of these attachments.

Another method is to press the splenic flexure laterally, superiorly, and posteriorly, then let go to evaluate how it feels during the return. Sidebending back and forth can aid in reaching the splenic flexure. A restriction will cause the return to be difficult, or change its direction.

Right lateral decubitus position

The patient reclines on the right side, head on a cushion or the bent right arm, left leg flexed, right leg extended. Standing behind the patient, push the rib cage anteriorly and inferiorly with the right hand, and use the fingers of the left hand to test different fibers of the left phrenicocolic ligament as above, and to evaluate potential restrictions.

In either of these two positions, you can ask the patient to slowly exhale deeply. With the fingers of your subcostal hand, create a support on the upper part of the descending colon and then the left part of the transverse colon, just in front of the splenic flexure. When the patient exhales, the splenic flexure moves superiorly and later-ally. Your supports permit evaluation of distensibility of the fibers of the left phrenico-colic ligament.

TEST OF THE SPLEEN ITSELF

As explained above, it is very difficult to differentiate between the spleen and its neighboring organs. Our goal here is really to look for resistance when structures in this area are mobilized superiorly and laterally. This pushes them into the "cradle" of the spleen formed by the superior surface of the left phrenicocolic ligament, near the spleen's inferior pole.

The patient is seated and bent forward. Place your hands exactly as you did for the test of the left phrenicocolic ligament, or place the fingers of both hands in the anterior left subcostal position.

Go past the splenic flexure and compress the structures in this area superiorly, posteriorly, and laterally toward the spleen. Change the location of your hands slightly several times, sometimes pressing in a medial direction to evaluate the difference in mobility and tissue resistance between the spleen itself and the gastrophrenic ligament.

Be careful not to force penetration of your fingers during this test. If you cause muscle contraction and pain, evaluation is impossible.

To increase the penetration of your fingers in the direction of the spleen during the test, sidebend the patient's torso to the left and keep it flexed forward. After position-ing your hands, rotate the torso to the right to draw the spleen toward your fingers.

TEST OF LEFT TRIANGULAR LIGAMENT OF THE LIVER

This test was described in our previous books, and is reviewed here because of the importance of this ligament in post-traumatic syndromes, and its relationship to the speen.

The left edge of the liver is easily palpable. It is anterior to the stomach, and is firm, almost hard. Its close relationship with the pericardium and diaphragm make it vulnerable to forces of collision, which tend to be focused on the left part of the thorax as explained above.

The left triangular ligament links the left edge of the liver to the diaphragm. Its restriction affects parts of the left gastrophrenic and phrenicocolic ligaments, and creates mechanical stress on the left part of the transverse mesocolon, all of which relate to the spleen.

For the test of the left triangular ligament, the subject is seated, arms relaxed, hands resting on thighs. Standing behind the patient, with your right knee on the table, place the palm of your left hand on the anterior left rib cage at the level of the ninth and tenth costochondral joints. The pads of your left fingers are 5-6cm beneath the costal margin, and the fingers of your right hand are on the left midclavicular line, pointed toward the left nipple . The fingers of both hands are directed superiorly, posteriorly, and to the left. The left palm draws the ribs toward the right, relaxing the left rectus abdominis *(Fig. 5-65)*.

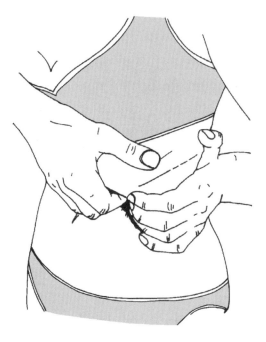

Fig. 5-65: Left triangular ligament test

While pressing with your fingers, forward bend the torso. Find the hard left edge of the liver, compress it superiorly, and assess its return.

The test is positive:

- if palpation of the left edge of the liver is sensitive or painful
- if it seems indurated, fibrous, and difficult to compress superiorly
- if its return is difficult or occurs along a different path.

TEST OF LEFT RIBS 8 THROUGH 12

Lack of lateral mobility of these ribs usually results from tensions in structures such as the transverse mesocolon and the left triangular phrenicocolic, gastrophrenic, and phrenicosplenic ligaments. Sometimes there are simply costovertebral restrictions, preventing normal costal movement.

In general, costal restrictions due to problems with the joints themselves give an impression of hardness during mobilization, whereas restrictions of visceral origin permit some limited movement.

For the test, the subject is supine, arms on the abdomen, legs extended. Standing to the right of the patient, place your right hand under the left eighth through tenth ribs, with your fingertips on the posterior angles. Your left hand is on the anterior aspect of the ribs *(Fig. 5-66)*.

Draw your right hand anteriorly and medially toward you. If there is a restriction of the liver, you will typically feel difficulty with this mobilization of the ribs. In contrast, with a left costovertebral restriction the ribs cannot move at all, even at the very beginning of mobilization. When there is a splenic restriction, mobilization is possible but feels restricted. Compare the two sides, remembering that the right side is slightly less mobile because of the liver.

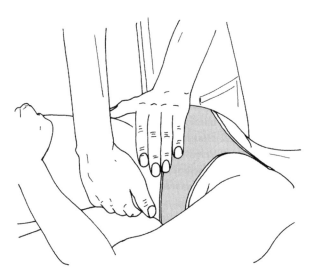

Fig. 5-66: Costosplenic test

Test of T8 through T10

These vertebrae correspond to the ribs described above. Mobility tests may reveal restrictions of the interapophyseal, costovertebral, or costotransverse articulations of the vertebrae or the posterior angles of the ribs.

The patient is seated, hands crossed behind the head, elbows raised and pointing forward. Stand behind the patient, place your right foot on the table, and your upper right forearm under the patient's elbows.

Press your left thumb successively against: the articular apophyses (one thumb's width lateral to the spinous process), costovertebral joints (two thumbs' distance), costotransverse joints (three thumbs' distance), and posterior costal angles (four or five thumbs' distance). Draw the spinal column and thorax in extension. With your thumb, push the interapophyseal, costovertebral, and costotransverse joints anterosuperiorly *(Fig. 5-67)*.

For the posterior costal angles, add right rotation to thoracic extension. Normally, the angle is easily mobilized anterolaterally *(Fig. 5-68)*. If there is articular restriction, you will feel a sensation of firmness, sometimes accompanied by sensitivity or pain from the very beginning of movement.

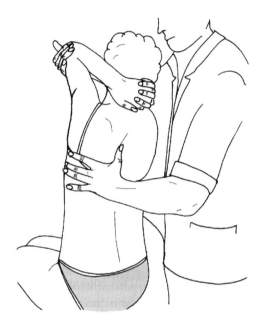

Fig. 5-67: Costovertebral test

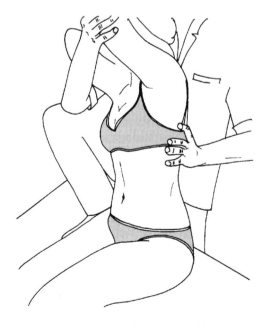

Fig. 5-68: Posterior angle test

Contraindications to Osteopathic Manipulation

Victims of significant trauma typically consult us after their hospitalization and completion of conventional medical tests. The "borderline" cases are the most difficult. You should never attempt osteopathic treatment following cervical trauma until x-rays, with an interpretive summary, are available. The following are the major contraindications to high-velocity, low-amplitude osteopathic techniques.

Signs of neurological deficits

Send the patient for complete neurological examination before beginning osteopathic treatment.

Paresthesia

This may indicate the presence of CNS or spinal injury, and also require a complete neurological examination.

Hypotension and hypertension

Slight post-traumatic hypotension may be due to internal hemorrhage. In this case, systolic tension is around 90cm H_2O. We have also seen cases of hypotension following leakage of CSF, which is very difficult to demonstrate.

Hypertension is less common, and is found after cranial trauma accompanied by cerebral compression due to increased CSF pressure.

Absence of tissue restriction

In some cases, post-traumatic pain is not accompanied by any articular or tissue restrictions. These patients should not be subjected to articular manipulation. The basic tenets of osteopathy require that we perform manipulation only upon vertebra or other joints that are restricted.

After trauma, there is a temporary "lull" during which the body has not yet reacted to its stresses, and restrictions have not yet formed. We must respect this prelesional state of calm and not cause any mechanical stress by manipulation.

Absence of symptoms

One of our many slogans is that "Better is the enemy of good." In other words, taking over the care of a patient who has no pain or signs of dysfunction is risky. There are two reasons for this:

- we may disturb compensation phenomena and provoke pain which was not previously expressed
- we may intervene just before the appearance of symptoms which would have appeared in any case. The patient concludes that our intervention triggered these symptoms. If you anticipate such a situation, it may be better to simply perform an osteopathic assessment without any treatment.

Recurrent discomfort

This may be due to vagotonia (hyperexcitability of the vagus nerve), which will, in theory, disappear without treatment. Vagotonic crises may be the expression of intense emotional reactions, osteoarticular problems of the cervical column, first rib (especially on the left), thoracic outlet, thoracic spine, or ribs (particularly at the T4/R4 level), preexisting cardiac problems, cerebral congestion, or diffuse micro-hemorrhages. All of these conditions require conventional medical workup before osteopathic treatment is attempted.

Repeated spontaneous dizziness

Craniocervical trauma frequently causes dizziness, but this is usually provoked by change of position. Spontaneous dizziness which appears at rest and without apparent cause is of greater concern. Dr. Emmanuel Cuzin (1992), of the ENT Department of the Pitié-Salpêtrière in Paris, describes two important types of spontaneous dizziness:

- the sensation of being on a merry-go-round indicates peripheral dizziness of the inner ear, and usually lasts for several hours
- the sensation of being drunk or on a boat indicates difficulty with equilibrium of central origin, which is usually much longer lasting.

Projectile vomiting

This can result from cranial hypertension, and requires immediate in-depth examination.

Troubles with vision

Cervical problems affect vision, but are only rarely severe enough to cause diplopia or hemianopia. When vision problems are significant, CNS or intraocular causes (e.g., detachment of the retina) are more likely.

Other miscellaneous contraindications

Be cautious if you encounter:

- unexplained fever, which may be related to serious visceral or internal cranial lesions
- a prostrate patient, who feels in danger. We have seen this in trauma victims with internal hemorrhage or preexisting neoplastic illness with no apparent relation to the accident.
- a patient with abnormal biochemical profiles, for example, high sedimentation rate and white cell count, indicating inflammation or infection.

Preexisting lesions present the greatest risk of error. Consider a patient who had an asymptomatic illness prior to her accident. Because of all the disturbances that trauma causes to the patient's physiology and psyche, it may cause her illness to "catch fire." She may believe that all the symptoms are due to the trauma. Without great vigilance on our part, a diagnostic error is almost inevitable.

We once had a patient who was unaware that she had an osseous cervical metastasis. She suffered slight cervical trauma in a rear-end auto collision. Two days later, she experienced severe cervicobrachial neuralgia, with nocturnal paroxysms. The severity of the symptoms relative to the low degree of trauma, in combination with painful palpation and mobility tests, caused us to suspect a nonmechanical lesion, which was later confirmed by x-ray.

Precautions to be Taken During Treatment

Observe a waiting period

It is prudent to wait about three weeks before beginning treatment of a trauma patient, for two reasons:

- the body needs time to adapt to and compensate for the forces of collision. The process of adaptation-compensation may be disturbed if you add further mechanical information. In fact, premature intervention can reinforce the effects of trauma.
- there is a latent period before certain symptoms appear, sometimes with a vengeance! If you intervene during this period, the patient may conclude that you are responsible for the new symptoms.

Request imaging studies

Osteopaths can develop an extremely sensitive touch and sometimes find lesions undetected by CT scan or MRI. However, the osteopathic touch is not infallible, and you may sometimes miss a fracture or preexisting lesion. Recall our case (described above) of the patient with an asymptomatic osseous cervical metastasis, who was rear-ended.

Measure blood pressure

Take the pressure systematically on both sides before beginning treatment. Do not manipulate a hypotensive patient if you do not know the reasons for his hypotension. A reactional vagotonia may occur following osteopathic treatment which increases hypotension. Imagine the effect on a patient who has blood pressure of 90mm Hg before treatment!

Vagotonic reactions occur primarily after vertebral manipulation, and are less common after craniosacral or visceral manipulation. Unilateral systolic hypotension almost always indicates the side with the restriction. At the end of the session, take the pressure again. It is a good sign if the pressure normalizes and the asymmetry disappears.

Be cautious with high-velocity, low-amplitude (HVLA) cervical manipulation

The cervical vertebrae are certainly the easiest to manipulate, for we can use all axes and directions. However, there is a risk that HVLA techniques will cause problems with the vertebral artery. We do direct HVLA cervical manipulation only after the following precautions:

- be familiar with the patient's reactivity
- first relax all the other tissue restrictions

- manipulate only cervical restrictions which are not secondary to other problems
- do not cause pain when applying tension prior to manipulation.

Support the patient's changes of position

After cranial or cervical trauma, the patient often feels dizzy when moving the head. When the patient is lying on his back, place a cushion high on the table and hold his head while he changes position such that the neck remains flexed and chin turned upward until the occiput contacts the cushion.

Before helping the patient get up, hold his head flexed for thirty seconds. This position reestablishes intracranial pressure and avoids orthostatic hypotension. These sorts of precautions increase the patient's confidence in your experience and abilities.

Explain possible post-manipulative reactions

These reactions are variable. When they do occur, it is typically after the first session, when the patient's body has not yet "learned" how to adapt to unfamiliar stimuli. Among the reactions which may follow osteopathic manipulation (mostly vagotonic) are:

- fatigue
- feeling of being bruised (this should be merely an impression!)
- disturbed cenesthesia (the sense of normal functioning of bodily organs)
- circadian variation in blood pressure
- stiffness upon awakening.

Chapter Six:
Treatment

Table of Contents

Treatment

General Remarks

As defined by Andrew Taylor Still, the founder of osteopathy, the goal of osteopathic treatment is to restore proper fluid circulation to the body. This is expressed in his well-known adage, "The rule of the artery is supreme." We effect changes in fluid circulation through tissue manipulation, whose goal is to restore the mobility of the structure to improve its function (Still: "Structure governs function.")

Effects of osteopathic treatment

Direct effects are obtained via the mechanoreceptors found in all tissues, including the:

- small short spinal muscles
- articular capsules and synovial membranes
- cranial membranes
- visceral ligaments and other attachments
- cartilage and bones.

Indirect effects are mediated by the CNS, which is stimulated by peripheral tissue proprioceptors. Reactions are produced in the following major systems:

- arterial
- cerebrospinal
- venolymphatic
- muscular/ligamentous
- psychoemotional.

Methods

Osteopathy is a *manual* form of medicine in which the practitioner's fingers seek out impaired tissues in order to relax them and restore their proper functioning.

Osteopathic treatment should be carried out by hand, and only by hand. In our view, the very foundations of osteopathic philosophy are betrayed if medications are prescribed in conjunction with manipulation.

To be optimally effective, osteopathy requires both precision and selectivity, that is, all techniques should be executed precisely and rapidly, using as little force as necessary. No more than three or four manipulations should be performed during a single visit. Furthermore, we recommend that there should be no more than three or four visits to treat a given problem. After all, osteopathic treatment aims to teach the body to cure itself. It is the patient who ultimately cures himself, not the practitioner.

We cannot finish this section without repeating Still's dictum on the osteopathic lesion which summarizes all the discussion above: *"Find it, fix it, and leave it alone!"*

Approach and terminology

Before getting into the details of treatment technique, we would like to clarify some important aspects of our approach to treatment and the related terminology. Many osteopathic textbooks from America describe manual diagnosis and treatment in terms of motion barriers. In this regard, direct techniques are those which go directly into and through motion barriers, while indirect techniques are those that are directed by a sense of ease that results from moving the involved tissues away from those barriers.

Our apporach to treatment for cranial and visceral lesions is somewhat different and is based on a clear understanding of the relevant anatomy and our skills in listening. We call a technique direct when it *directly* lengthens the restricted tissues. While this can be thought of as similar to techniques which engage and go through a motion barrier, our techniques are more concerned with stretching and releasing the tissues than with any particular barrier.

When we say that a technique is indirect, we are referring to something that is *listening-driven.* This means that the direction of forces applied by the practitioner are completely aligned with the direction of motion felt by listening. Depending on the tissues involved and the individual situation, these listening-driven forces may be in the direction of a barrier felt on motion testing, in the direction of ease when doing motion testing, or in a completely different direction. To perform these techniques with maximum efficacy, it is important not to confuse these approaches and terms.

Treatment

In this book, we describe certain osteopathic techniques which we have selected based on their originality and effectiveness. In actual practice, of course, we do not limit our treatment to these few techniques; nor should you. These are simply presented as a framework around which you can design your own treatment of trauma.

Manipulation of cranial bones and sutures

Following cranial trauma, forces of collision may be retained in the periosteum, bone, sutures, and membrane system. The goal of the following techniques is to restore the elasticity and distensibility of these structures in the skull. Traditionally, osteopaths have been more interested in sutural than osseous restrictions, but we believe this is an overly restrictive view. The bone itself must regain its initial compressibility and elasticity.

Coronal suture

The patient is supine, legs extended, hands resting on the chest.

DIRECT TECHNIQUE

Sitting behind the patient, place the heel of your dominant hand on the frontal, *immediately in front of the coronal suture*, with your middle finger along the sagittal axis. The occiput rests on your other palm, on the table.

With both arms flexed, push the frontal inferiorly and slightly anteriorly, as if you were trying to separate the edges of the coronal suture. Distensibility tests which you have performed previously enable you to focus the corrective pressure on the most restricted areas, which are often small areas of approximately 2cm in length.

Use a direct technique with significant pressure (up to 500g), but never cause discomfort or pain. Apply the pressure rhythmically, in synch with the patient's tissues, usually between five and ten cycles per minute. Your movement should be strong and slow, and four to five repetitions are usually sufficient.

INDIRECT TECHNIQUE

In the same position, while beginning to apply tension to the two edges of the coronal suture, exert your force in the direction of listening. For those who are accustomed to traditional osteopathic functional techniques which involve only an "intention" of movement, we should emphasize that these techniques involve more gross movement, similar to that of significant stretching or a thrust.

When you actively follow the direction of listening, your movement seems long and often curved. Repeat the movement four or five times, and retest the suture to evaluate reestablishment of its distensibility. After successful sutural correction, local listening should be negative.

Some patients respond best to rapidly executed manipulation, while others require a slower rhythm. You will need to determine the optimal speed for your maneuvers, depending on the particular patient.

Petro-occipital junction

BILATERAL PETRO-OCCIPITAL DISIMPACTION

This technique is useful following whiplash. It helps restore good mobility to the base of the skull and gives the occiput back its freedom within the PRM.

The patient is supine. Hold your hands cupped, with the patient's head in the palms. Your fifth fingers join on the occipital median line, coming as close as possible to the posterior arc of C1, or the foramen magnum. The third and fourth fingers are placed laterally, with their tips as far as possible in the direction of the foramen magnum. The index fingers are immediately behind the mastoid process, in front of the occipitomastoid suture. The thumbs are in front of the index fingers, behind the ear *(Fig. 6-1)*.

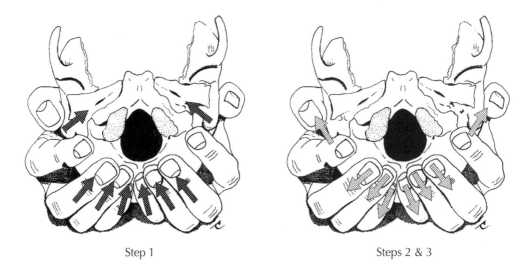

Step 1   Steps 2 & 3

Fig. 6-1: Bilateral petroccipital disimpaction

Step one. The third, fourth, and fifth ("occipital") fingers push the occiput an-teriorly during the craniosacral expansion phase (circumferential forward translation of the occiput), while the index fingers and thumbs press the temporals medially. This temporarily increases compression.

Step two. The occipital fingers try to push the basilar part of the occiput superiorly while maintaining their anterior movement. This disengagement of the basilar occiput is obtained indirectly, by trying to bend the occiput according to its large radius of curva-ture, between the pads and heels of the hands. During this time, the index fingers and thumbs support the temporals.

Step three. The index fingers and thumbs draw the temporals anteriorly and later-ally, while the occipital fingers pull the occipital squama posteriorly in a movement of circumferential translation. This disengagement is done with respect for the tension and points of attachment. They do not all yield at the same rate, and should not be forced.

Unilateral petro-occipital disimpaction

If mobility is not completely restored with the bilateral technique, we can focus our manipulation on one side of the restriction. This unilateral technique utilizes the same parameters, but with a different handhold.

Sit at the patient's head, which is slightly inclined toward the unrestricted side. One hand is on the affected temporal, using the classic five-finger hold:

- the zygomatic process is between the thumb and index finger
- the middle finger is in the external auditory canal
- the ring finger is on the tip of the mastoid process
- the little finger is on the mastoid base.

The occipital hand is almost perpendicular to the axis of the occiput, with the index close to the foramen magnum, and the fingertips placed parallel to the petro-occip-ital suture *(Fig. 6-2).*

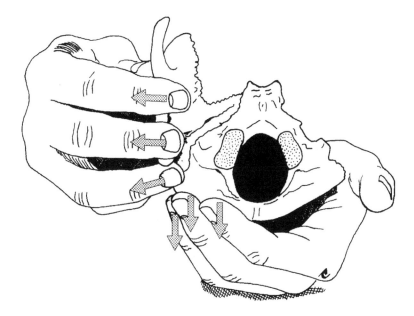

Fig. 6-2: Unilateral petroccipital disimpaction: steps 2 & 3

Step one: The fingers of the occipital hand push anteriorly, while those of the temporal hand exert compression against the basilar occiput.

Step two: The occipital hand increases flexion and pulling of the bone, to disengage the basilar occiput superiorly.

Step three: The temporal hand draws the temporal laterally and anteriorly, while the occipital hand draws the occiput posteriorly and laterally in the opposite direction.

Other sutures (squamoparietal)

In contrast to the coronal suture, techniques for other sutures combine work on osseous elasticity with sutural manipulations. We will use the squamoparietal suture as an example.

The patient is in lateral decubitus position, head resting with the treated side up. Place the thenar eminence of one hand on the parietal to push it medially and superiorly, the other on the temporal to direct it inferiorly and laterally. Your primary goal is to separate the edges of the squamoparietal suture *(Fig. 6-3).*

Direct technique

The upper parts of the thenar eminences are focused on the sutures, while the lower parts focus on parietal and temporal osseous elasticity. The corrective effect is divided in two movements which become joined at the end.

- The first movement draws the palms medially, as if the parietal and temporal were going in the direction of the table.
- The second separates the temporal from the parietal.

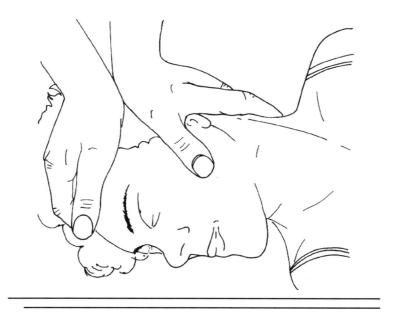

Fig. 6-3: Squamoparietal osteosutural manipulation

The work on osseous elasticity is essential. This is a powerful movement but should not be unpleasant or painful. Five to six repetitions should suffice.

INDIRECT TECHNIQUE

This consists of directing the corrective pushes in the direction of sutural listening *while taking osseous listening into account*. This is quite difficult.

At first, you should take the direction given by osseous listening into account before following the sutural listening. To do this, you must first directly compress and decompress the osseous part several times to stimulate the direction of listening.

Craniofacial membranous system

This technique, when properly executed, achieves excellent results in young children after only one or two sessions. It is important to restore craniofacial mobility following trauma or fetal displacement which cause residual deformations or restrictions of the palate.

PALATE

Direct technique

The patient is supine, arms at the sides, legs extended. Face the right shoulder (or left shoulder, if you are left-handed) and place the tip of the crooked index finger of your dominant hand on the anterior or lateral part of the palatine process of the maxilla, depending upon the restriction. Your other hand is on the forehead as a stabilizing force. Exert traction anteriorly and slightly superiorly with the dominant hand, as if trying to separate the maxilla from the skull *(Fig. 6-4)*.

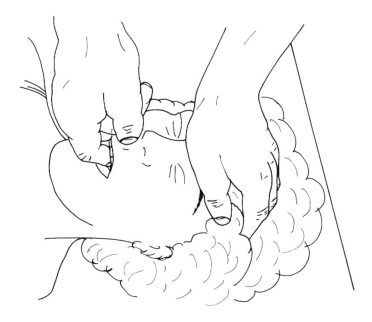

Fig. 6-4: Roof of the mouth, direct manipulation

Perform progressive traction in an anterior direction. If the tissues bring your finger somewhat laterally, follow that movement. Never put pressure on the teeth! They are sometimes weakly set in their sockets because of trauma, osteoporosis, or cavities.

The direct technique permits relaxation of the anterior attachments of the dura mater through the falx cerebri.

Indirect technique

This technique is essential for correcting craniofacial restrictions. After drawing the palate superiorly and anteriorly, you gently relax the traction, and then allow it to follow the direction of listening.

The indirect technique more effectively corrects sequelae of trauma, fetal mal-positioning, and certain orthodontic problems related to slightly curved or oblique osteomembranous restrictions that occur during growth.

Four to six repetitions should suffice. To confirm the effect of the correction, retest the craniofacial system by listening. There should no longer be a local listening. This technique is also useful for sinusitis and chronic headaches.

MAXILLAE

The techniques we use for the maxillae treat not only the sutural articulations but also the cranial/facial/maxillary membranous system. The patient is supine. Place the thumb and index finger of your dominant hand on the two sides of the maxillae, just posterior to the base of the zygomatic processes. To obtain sufficient traction, it is neces-sary that the thumb and index finger be placed inside the mouth directly on these pillars. Be careful not to put any pressure on the teeth themselves. The thumb and middle finger (or index finger for children) of the other hand press on the frontal at the level of the temples, just above the sphenofrontal sutures *(Fig. 6-5)*.

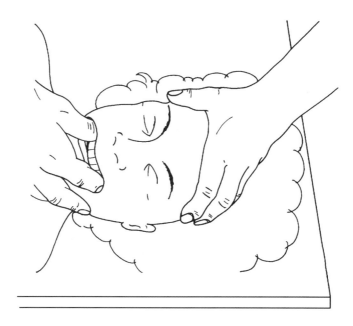

Fig. 6-5: Craniofacial membranous manipulation

Indirect technique

We prefer the indirect to the direct technique, as the latter may increase tension on the membranes and cause headaches.

Most of the time, the frontal and maxillae move in opposite directions during listening. With your fingers, execute these lateral movements four or five times, until you feel the direction induced by the listening decrease and stop. This maneuver confers real mobility, and the technique is surprisingly effective if your manipulations are performed in the direction of listening.

Direct technique

The direct technique can be used by highly skilled practitioners when there is an absence of mobility associated with hardened membranes. It is most commonly used for chronic sinusitis and headaches, or severe post-traumatic sequelae.

Dura mater manipulations

Stretching/listening of the longitudinal sinus

While this is a technique performed in the direction of the longitudinal sinus, it's use should not be limited to conditions of the venous sinuses. In fact, the main purpose of this technique is to stretch the dura *(Fig. 6-6)*.

The patient is supine, legs extended, hands on the chest. Seated behind the patient, with your elbows flexed, place the hypothenar eminence of your dominant hand just anterior to the lambda (where the lambdoid and sagittal sutures meet at the posterior fontanel). Your middle finger is placed over the sagittal suture. The palm of your other hand holds the occiput.

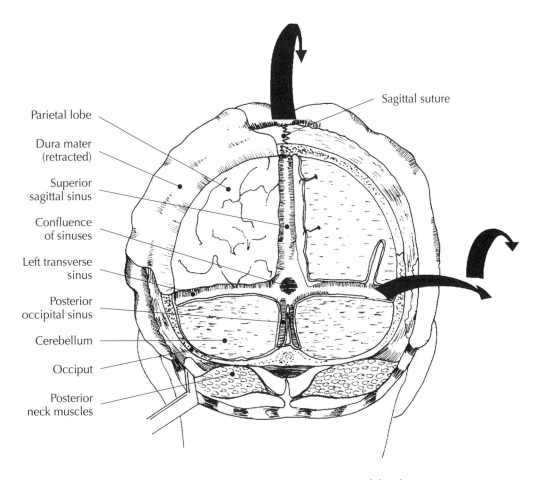

Parietal lobe

Dura mater
(retracted)

Superior
sagittal sinus

Confluence
of sinuses

Left transverse
sinus

Posterior
occipital sinus

Cerebellum

Occiput

Posterior
neck muscles

Sagittal suture

Fig. 6-6: Anteroposterior and lateral manipulation of the dura mater

DIRECT TECHNIQUE

This consists of pushing anteriorly and slightly caudad along the direction of the sagittal suture. It is important to have your elbows flexed to produce a movement which comes from your entire upper arm and body. This technique can affect the bones, dura mater, and falx cerebri. Significant restrictions (usually from trauma or fetal malpositioning) can cause the movement to vary slightly from the sagittal plane, obliquely toward one of the shoulders.

INDIRECT TECHNIQUE

This is used slightly less often than other techniques. It restores a lack of sagittal distensibility of the skull caused by restrictions of the dura mater, falx cerebelli, or tentorium cerebelli. Restrictions which require this technique in order to be released are usually not completely sagittal. The movement induced by listening is often divided in two directions:

- the first directs the palm in the direction of one of the acromioclavicular joints. This is an "intention" of a movement.

- the second directs the palm posteriorly and deeply in the direction of the ipsilateral sternoclavicular joint.

With your eyes closed, the movements you are executing should seem smooth and unbroken, even with the several changes of direction.

Stretching/ listening of the lateral sinus

The patient is in lateral decubitus position, head turned in the direction opposite from the sinus to be treated. Standing behind the patient, place a palm against the posterior edge of the mastoid process and push it anteriorly, inferiorly, and slightly laterally *(Fig. 6-7)*, taking into account the direction of the lateral sinus. The other palm creates an active counterforce on the occiput, midway between the external protuberance and the parietal.

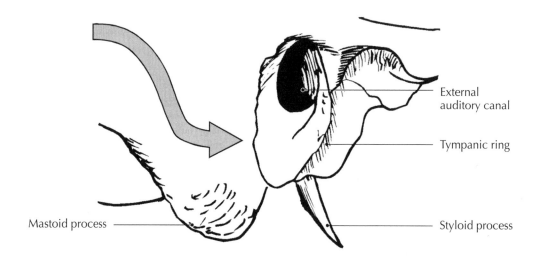

Fig. 6-7: Direction of stretching of the lateral sinus

Perform these maneuvers in a manner that does not involve the spinal cord. The slightest pain is a signal to change the position of the nape of the neck. At the point of strongest pressure, release the pressure slightly and follow the direction of tissue listening. Four or five repetitions are sufficient.

Combination techniques for cranial dura mater

TENTORIUM CEREBELLI TECHNIQUE

This technique, particularly effective when one side of the tentorium is tense, utilizes the distinctive feature of reciprocal tension between the spinal dura mater and intracranial membranes. When there is sidebending in the spine, this releases neurological structures on the side of the spinal concavity, as well as the tentorium. On the convex side, there is increased tension of the neurological elements which constrains the tentorium.

Sit next to the patient's head. This technique has two possible approaches:

- asymmetrical approach: one hand is underneath the occiput, the other holds the treated temporal bone with the five-finger hold
- symmetrical approach: the hands are crossed underneath the occiput, with the thumbs and thenar eminences along the upper mastoid portion of the two temporal bones.

The first step is to relax the tentorium by:

- internal rotation of the temporal bone on the side being treated, even lightly pressing it against the occiput, in order to increase relaxation
- sidebending the spine toward the treated side. You help the patient flex the ipsilateral hip and knee by taking hold of the ankle on that side, and tilting the cervical spine toward the treated side *(Fig. 6-8)*.

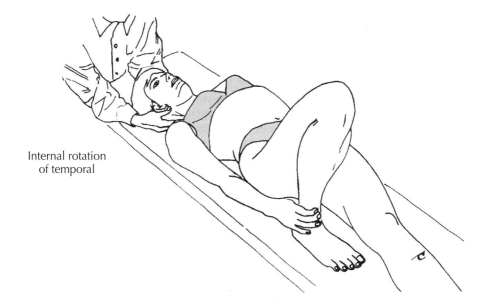

Internal rotation
of temporal

Fig. 6-8: Tentorium cerebelli technique, step 1: relaxation

Wait until you feel a release of tension under your fingers. By closing your eyes when this release occurs, you will feel the temporal bone begin to rotate externally.

The second step of the technique is to stretch the treated side of the tentorium by:

- external rotation of the temporal bone
- sidebending the spine in the opposite direction, by asking the patient to extend the previously flexed leg and then sidebending the cervical spine in the opposite direction, assisted by slight anterior flexion of the head. Carry out this stretching gently three or four times. By paying close attention to the tension of the tissues, you can clearly feel how much stretching can be accomplished with each repetition. If you are doing the technique correctly, the amplitude will increase with each repetition *(Fig. 6-9)*.

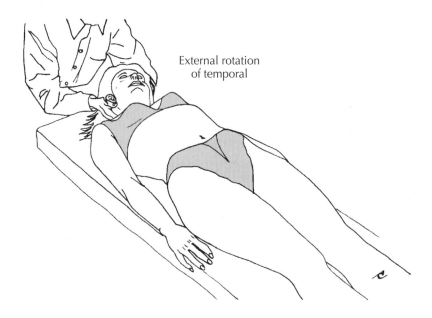

External rotation
of temporal

Fig. 6-9: Tentorium cerebelli technique, step 2: stretching

FALX CEREBRI AND FALX CEREBELLI

Stretching or shortening of these intracranial falciform structures is achieved utilizing antagonistic tension between the cranial and spinal segments of the dura mater.

Stretching the spinal column shortens the spinal cord, which reduces encephalic pressure on the tentorium. The latter causes release of the falx cerebri, which becomes "shortened," and increased tension of the falx cerebelli, which becomes "stretched." Conversely, flexion of the spine increases pressure on the tentorium, with consequent tension of the falx cerebri (which is pulled downward) and relaxation of the falx cerebelli (which is slightly shortened). See Fig. 2-27 in Chapter 2.

To release and shorten the falx cerebri, you reduce the anteroposterior and vertical diameters of the skull, while simultaneously guiding the cervical spine carefully in traction. Conversely, to stretch the falx cerebri, which you can visualize as a "fan," you lengthen its peripheral insertions while flexing the cervical spine.

OBELION

The obelion is a craniometric point near the lambda, on the sagittal suture between the parietal foramina. We have noticed in dissections a peculiar fibrous disposition related to the obelion, which is almost always present on the falx cerebri and falx cerebelli.

When looking at slide sections of falx cerebri one sees, among the other distribution systems of dura mater fibers, two major categories of longitudinal fibers:

- those issuing from the area of frontal insertion, ending in the anterior parietal bone, in the vicinity of the posterior obelion

• those issuing from the area of occipital insertion, ending in the posterior parietal bone, in the vicinity of the anterior obelion.

In this fibrous distribution, the obelion is at the intersection of what could be called an anterior horizontal hemifalx and a posterior vertical hemifalx *(Fig. 6-10)*.

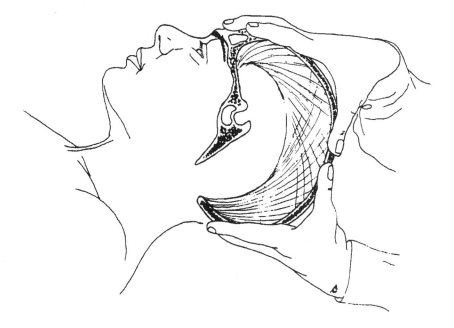

Fig. 6-10: Obelion: test and treatment

The obelion, to us, seems to be the center of equilibrium of the sagittal dura mater structures. It enables us to localize more precisely losses of elasticity of the falx cerebri and falx cerebelli. One can investigate two directions of fibers by "circling" an area in the obelion-nasion (landmark where intranasal and nasofrontal sutures meet) and comparing its deformability and malleability with that of an area in the obelion-opisthion (midpoint of posterior border of the foramen magnum).

You can specifically place the most restricted part of the obelion in traction, and apply a recoil technique when releasing the traction. You can also work on the obelion as a point of maximal density of the falces, and apply to it a compression listening in the direction of the sphenobasilar symphysis.

Spinal dura mater

Suboccipital traction monitoring

The patient is in supine position, arms at the sides, legs extended. Place both palms underneath the occiput with the two index fingers, one on top of the other, on the inferior occipital line just above the atlas. Use these fingers to exert traction on the occiput while listening (in general, superiorly and slightly anteriorly) *only during the expansion phase of craniosacral motion.* During the relaxation phase, ease off on the traction *(Fig. 6-11)*.

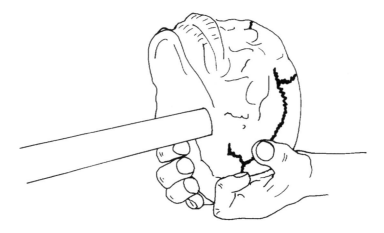

Fig. 6-11: Traction with listening on the cylinder of the dura mater

Carry out this maneuver with eyes closed to get a feeling of slow, progressive, unending movement. Sometimes the first movement felt is in the longitudinal axis, followed by movements along oblique or lateral axes. Stay alert to catch these subtle changes in direction. Too much resistance to stretching of the occiput means that you have not followed the direction of listening, or that the patient is not in craniosacral flexion phase. When the technique is performed correctly, you will clearly feel improved occipital/vertebral distensibility, and an impression of intraspinal release.

Stretching the lower part of the dura mater sleeve (T9/sacrum)

The patient position is the same as above. Place your cephalad hand under the T8/9 region. Keep in mind the anatomic narrowing of the spinal canal at T9. The corresponding narrowing of the spinal dura mater enables us to differentiate two distinct zones.

Hold the spinous process of T9 with the index and middle fingers of your cephalad hand. With your caudad hand, exert traction on the sacrum in a pedad direction. Support at T9 is important. Act as if it were a ring, threaded on the dura mater cylinder, that you are trying to slip on superiorly and anteriorly.

This is a "structural" tissue technique. Release is obtained by creating strong traction between your two hands. The goal is to mobilize, stretch, and (if possible) release the dura mater in the vertebral canal.

VARIATION

With the patient in prone position, place your crossed hands as a support for T9 and the sacrum. With the crossed position you obtain more force, and a balance of depth and stretching.

This technique is good for treating the painful sequelae of a spinal tap or peridural anesthesia.

Stretching the upper part of the dura mater sleeve (T9/occiput)

This technique uses the same principles as the preceding one. This time, the cephalad hand holds the occiput and draws it superiorly, while the thumb and index of the caudad hand grasp the T9 spinous process.

Stretching both ends of the spinal dura mater

There are two possible methods, described below.

SUPINE

With the patient in the position shown in Fig. 6-12:

- your occipital hand is pronated and approaches the occiput contralaterally, with the fingers directed toward the vertex while following the axis of cranial symmetry as closely as possible
- your sacral hand also follows the symmetry of the bone. The inferolateral angles of the sacrum rest on the thenar and hypothenar eminences.

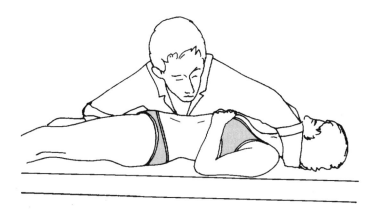

Fig. 6-12: Stretching via the ends of the spinal dura mater in supine position

Gently flex the sacrum and slightly extend the occiput on C1. While maintaining this engagement of the two ends of the spinal dura, add a slight tension between your hands *(Fig. 6-13)*.

Mobilize the two ends with an eccentric gliding movement, that is, in a superior direction for the occipital hand and inferior direction for the sacral hand. Induce maximal elasticity of the spinal dura mater and you will feel the limit pushed further back each time. Repeat gently but firmly, in a rhythmic manner, until you feel a release.

PRONE

The patient lies prone, forehead resting on the table or on the hands. Cross your arms, and place one hand on the occiput, the other on the sacral base *(Fig. 6-14)*. Stretch the dura mater in the direction of listening, separating your points of support from each other. One drawback of this powerful approach is that it presses the patient's face against the table, unless you are fortunate enough to have a table with a hole cut out for the face.

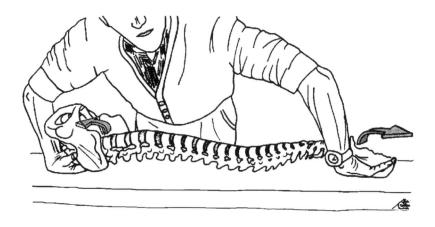

Fig. 6-13: Stretching via the ends of the spinal dura mater in supine position (skeletal view)

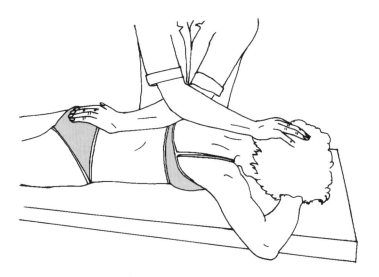

Fig. 6-14: Stretching via the ends of the spinal dura mater in prone position

Stretching/listening of the cervicobrachial plexus

The cervicobrachial plexus and its surrounding tissues have many important relationships, and this technique is useful for most problems of the thoracic inlet and upper extremities.

The patient is supine, legs extended, arms at the sides. Stand at the patient's head, with the middle or index finger of one hand on the indented palpable interlamellar cervical region, as shown in Fig. 5-25 in Chapter 5. Place the thumb of your other hand on the most sensitive part of the cervicobrachial plexus, between the anterior edge of the trapezius and the clavicle. The cervical finger lightly compresses the indented interlamellar region by stretching in the direction of listening, while the thumb on the nerves performs stretching/listening *(Fig. 6-15)*.

It is as if your thumb were trying to stretch the nerve projections laterally, anter-

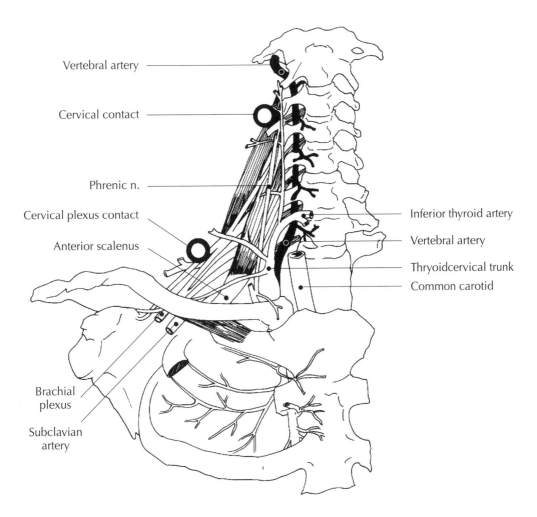

Vertebral artery

Cervical contact

Phrenic n.

Cervical plexus contact

Anterior scalenus

Inferior thyroid artery

Vertebral artery

Thryoidcervical trunk

Common carotid

Brachial plexus

Subclavian artery

Fig. 6-15: Stretching of the cervicobrachial plexus

iorly, and inferiorly. This is not a pure movement, but rather a combination of changes in movement in the general direction described above. Your two hands have to work synergistically with each other. With your eyes closed, you should have a sensation of unending movement of your thumb. The maneuver is complete when you have the impression of a cord loosening.

Once this part of the plexus has been released, the nerve can be followed distally. For example, you can move to the ipsilateral side of the patient, placing your cephalad hand under the clavicle and your caudad hand in the axilla. Once you have found the nerve with each hand (usually easiest using the thumbs), work your hands together as described above until you feel a release. This type of technique can be continued down the arm to the wrist, if necessary.

Remember while you are working that the goal of this technique is to get the nerve to glide more smoothly. Keep that smooth gliding motion in mind while working and you will avoid the problem of being too heavy-handed.

Indications

- *Unequal dura mater tension.* This technique can lead to the establishment of equal tensions along the longitudinal axis of the dural tube.

- *Sciatica.* While it may seem odd to treat this area for sciatica, it is a good illustration of how the body is all interconnected. It is common for restrictions and congestion of the lumbosacral plexus to be accompanied by similar problems of the cervicobrachial plexus, as the congested nerve roots lose their distensibility, and, through the perineurium, transfer this tension to the other end of the dural tube. For this reason, stretching of the cervicobrachial plexus indirectly leads to relaxation of the periradicular dura mater tension around the sciatic nerve.

- *Cervicobrachial neuralgia.* With this type of neuralgia, there is inflammation with edema and venous stasis at the foraminal level. The radicular sleeve is restricted and loses it ability to elongate. Mobilizing the cervicobrachial plexus reduces this congestion, restores mobility, and significantly reduces pain.

- *Autonomic connections.* The cervicobrachial plexus has many anastomoses with both the parasympathetic and sympathetic nervous systems. By releasing restrictions here you may affect:

  – on the left side, the heart, bronchi, esophagus, stomach, spleen, and gallbladder
  – on the right side, the bronchi, liver, pylorus, duodenum, and pancreas.

Sacral dura mater

Seated position

We describe here only the indirect technique, which is the most effective.

The patient is seated on the table, with both hands behind the neck. Standing behind the patient, with your right foot on the table, place your right forearm on your right knee, with both the patient's elbows resting on your upper arm. Hold the sacrum with your left palm, with your middle and index fingers on the sacrococcygeal joint and coccyx *(Fig. 6-16)*. Follow the movements of sacrococcygeal listening, exaggerating them, while also following the general listening of the body (which is sometimes different).

The movements felt and performed usually occur in several steps:

- an initial movement of the coccyx relative to the sacrum
- a movement of the sacrum relative to the bladder and lumbar spine
- finally, a global movement of the entire body.

At the beginning of the movement, let the entire weight of the body rest on your hand. To stretch the dura mater, you must transmit the global listening of the body at the sacral level, as well as the sacrococcygeal local listening which reflects the dura mater tension.

Do this about twelve times until you feel a local release of the sacrum and a cessation of global listening. This many repetitions are necessary because the structures involved are very strong.

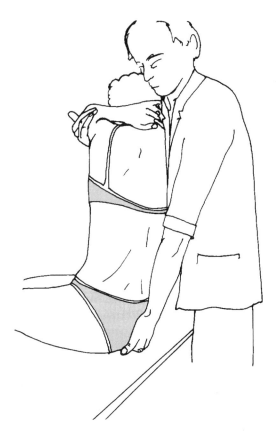

Fig. 6-16: Sacral dura mater manipulation in seated position

Supine position: intrarectal techniques

We have previously discussed the internal sacrococcygeal manipulations, which involve primarily the anterior, posterior, and lateral articular ligaments (Barral and Mercier, 1988 and Barral, 1989). The technique described here involves the inferior end of the common posterior vertebral ligament, periosteum, and sacrodural ligament.

The common posterior vertebral ligament descends from the occiput anterior to the dura mater. At its inferior end, after the lumbosacral joint, it thins out until it disappears around the first coccygeal segment. It is at this level that the sacrodural ligament of Trolard becomes restricted, connecting the dura mater to the anterior wall of the sacral canal.

Some researchers believe that the sacrodural ligament serves normally as an inferior longitudinal tensor of the dura mater. Our own dissections have not entirely convinced us of this. However, following trauma to the lower body, this rather thin ligament may thicken and shorten until it has an effect on the dura mater, creating an abnormal longitudinal tension.

The common posterior vertebral ligament is joined by connective tissue tracts to the dura mater and adheres closely to the vertebral disks. Therefore, bulging disk problems can affect the dura mater, and vice versa.

For these techniques the patient is prone, forehead resting on the hands. The index finger of your dominant hand penetrates deeply through the rectum, reaching as close as possible to the second sacral segment. The thumb of this hand rests on the posterior part of the sacrum, while the palm of the other hand exerts counterforce at the S1-S2 level.

DIRECT TECHNIQUE

The intrarectal index finger is placed against the smooth surface of the sacrum, from which it is separated by the presacral aponeurosis. The coccyx rests on the meta-carpophalangeal joint of the finger. In the first step, the distal phalanx pushes the second sacral segment posteriorly and slightly inferiorly. This is not really a movement, rather a static push in the direction of the correction.

In the second step, the entire index finger draws the sacrum in an anterior swing movement up to the sacrococcygeal joint. The sacral promontory is directed anteriorly, while the coccyx is raised posteriorly. The palm of the external hand exerts active counterforce by pushing S1-S2 anteriorly.

The general movement of the sacrum between the two ilia, combined with movement of the coccyx, permits an effect on the dura mater. Work with your entire body, both arms flexed. These movements should be powerful but completely painless.

INDIRECT TECHNIQUE

As usual, you begin with the direct technique, relax it slightly during the movement, and begin again following the direction given by local listening. The indirect technique permits you to refine the corrective maneuver, adding slight sidebending or rotation to the direct sagittal mobilization. Four or five repetitions should suffice.

Presacral aponeurosis and periosteum: intrarectal technique

This technique indirectly affects the dura mater and is very effective for sequelae of sacrococcygeal falls. With the end of the intrarectal index finger slightly crooked, seek out irregularities or striations on the anterior surface of the sacrum. In principle, this surface should be totally smooth in a person who has not been a victim of trauma. In cases of sacrococcygeal trauma, digital palpation enables you to feel actual "grooves" at the osteoperiostal level. Press the pad of the index on these (often painful) grooves and carry out small longitudinal and transverse movements in the direction of listening, as if you were trying to erase the grooves while stretching the presacral aponeurosis.

This technique requires a dozen manipulations performed rather slowly, as the structures involved are strong. The technique can be effective for urogenital problems as well as the sequelae of sacrococcygeal trauma.

Stretching of the external rotators of the hip

Stretching of these muscles is always indicated following trauma. These techniques are particularly effective in cases in which the entire spinal column and pelvis have been affected. Other indications are sciatica, urinary stress incontinence, pelvic congestion, and lower limb pathology. Good release of the lateral hip rotators has a beneficial effect on the sacrum, coccyx, lumbosacral plexus, arcuate pubic ligament, femoral head, urogenital system, and lower limbs.

The patient is supine, hands crossed on the chest, leg on the treated side flexed, other leg extended. Sit on a stool facing the treated hip.

Direct technique

First method. We will use the right hip as an example. Place two or three fingers of your left hand inside the intertrochanteric line, close to the trochanteric fossa. Keep the fingers flat to avoid irritating this sensitive region. Your right hand grasps the anterior surface of the knee to draw the thigh in external rotation and abduction, which helps you better position your fingers on the posteromedial portion of the greater trochanter *(Fig. 6-17).*

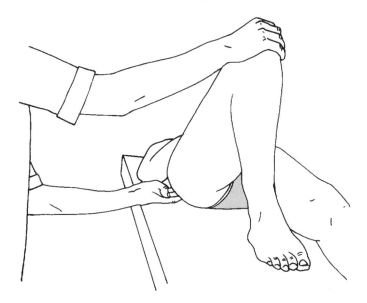

Fig. 6-17: Stretching of the external hip rotators (1st method)

Stretch the greater trochanter posterolaterally, with slight external rotation, while flexing and abducting the hip. Next, draw the thigh in internal rotation, adduction, and extension. Maintain these tractions until the lower leg rests on the table.

Second method. For heavy patients who are difficult to mobilize, place the treated thigh and leg in external rotation, abduction, and flexion, with the foot resting on the opposite thigh. Place two to three fingers of both hands on top of one another, under the posteromedial part of the greater trochanter, to perform posterolateral traction, as above.

Ask the patient to stretch out her leg, while sliding the foot along the medial aspect of the opposite leg, until the treated leg rests on the table. In this way, the treated leg passively executes the same movement that you actively direct with the first method: internal rotation, adduction, and extension.

Indirect technique

The indirect version of the first method above consists of stretching the greater trochanter posterolaterally, and slightly relaxing the traction to follow the direction of listening. Meanwhile, the other hand holds the knee to mobilize the treated thigh, also following the direction of listening.

In the indirect version of the second method, since the leg is being mobilized by the patient, you follow the direction of listening only with the subtrochanteric fingers.

The indirect techniques allow more precision in stretching the lateral rotators.

Ischiofemoral stretching

This is an important complement to stretching of the lateral hip rotators. Indications for use include sciatica, pelvic trauma, and problems of the urogenital system or lower limbs. The patient is in the same position. Stand up, facing the treated hip.

We will again take a right-sided restriction as an example. Place the fingers of your right hand under the anteromedial part of the right ischiopubic ramus, engaging it well. Place your left palm on the lateral side of the flexed knee on the treated side, and draw the femur in maximal adduction, with the knee ending up above the other knee *(Fig. 6-18)*. Next, draw the thigh in extension, while maintaining good adduction. This technique is beneficial for the lateral hip rotators (particularly the quadratus femoris), the sacrotuberous and sacrospinal ligaments, and perineal muscles.

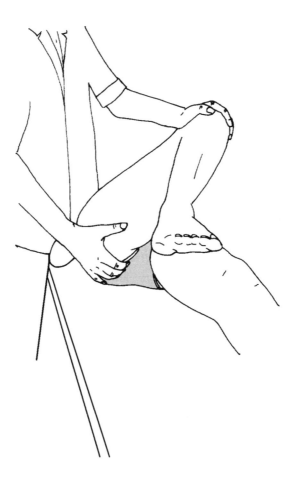

Fig. 6-18: Ischiofemoral stretching

Stretching of the lumbosacral plexus

The patient is supine, hands on the abdomen, hip and knee on the treated side flexed, other leg resting on the table.

Direct technique

First method: Sit on the table, in front of the flexed knee. The goal is to stretch the lumbosacral plexus via the sciatic nerve. For the right sciatic nerve, place your left index finger flat in the ischiofemoral groove *(Fig. 6-19)*. Your right hand is on the antero-lateral part of the knee to slightly flex the thigh.

Bring your left finger up to the piriformis muscle. Continue to flex the thigh while keeping the index finger pressed against the nerve in the groove, so as to stretch the sciatic nerve toward the thigh and slightly laterally.

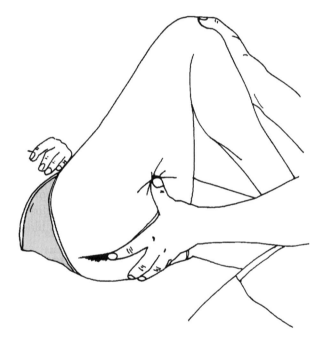

Fig. 6-19: Stretching of the lumbosacral plexus via the sciatic nerve

While maintaining traction of the sciatic nerve, at first laterally rotate and abduct the hip, then switch to extension, internal rotation, and adduction until the leg rests on the table.

The difficult part of this technique is mobilizing the hip while continuing to simultaneously press and stretch the index finger against the groove, particularly during the extension/adduction/internal rotation phase.

Second method: For heavy patients, sit facing the greater trochanter of the treated side, and place the foot against the medial surface of the opposite thigh. Press both index fingers, on top of one another, in the groove against the sciatic nerve. Maintain this pressure while stretching the sciatic nerve toward the thigh. Ask the patient to slowly slide the foot along the leg until the treated leg is completely extended.

It is essential to place the two index fingers well anteriorly and medially so as not to lose contact with the femur. This requires concentration and appropriate force.

Indirect technique

The index finger of your dominant hand presses on the sciatic nerve in the groove, while stretching it toward the thigh, following the direction of listening. Often, the listening leads the index finger medially, with slight internal rotation at the completion of stretching.

Indications

- *Dura mater restrictions.* This technique is used to reestablish inferior longitudinal equilibrium tension of the dura mater after trauma, sequelae of fetal malposition, or scoliosis.
- *Sciatica.* Stretching of the sciatic nerve and lumbosacral plexus releases the mobility of the radicular sleeve, and reduces congestion from periradicular venous stasis. The sciatic nerve technique can give immediate, noticeable gains in the straight leg raising test.
- *Cervicobrachial neuralgia.* All radicular inflammations involve tension in the perineurium and adjacent dura mater, which may be reflected on the ipsilateral extremity at the other end of the body. Through release of reciprocal tension by stretching of the sciatic nerve, you can reduce inflammation of both the cervicobrachial and lumbosacral plexuses.
- *Genital system.* Pelvic pain of genital origin may be reduced through the lumbosacral plexus and, indirectly, the hypogastric plexus.

Comments

Whenever someone has sciatica, be sure to do this technique on *both* sides. This is due to the reciprocal tension relationship between both sides of the lower dura. Otherwise, your efforts will have less than optimal effect and the problem can easily recur. If working on the affected side does not improve the situation, work on the other side to get a release through this reciprocal tension.

In extremely acute cases of sciatica, this technique cannot be done, as the nerve in the ischiofemoral groove is too "hot" to be touched. One way around this is to start the technique lower down on the posterior thigh, between the biceps femoris and semimembranosus muscles. To do this, sit at the feet of the supine patient and have them flex the hip and knee of the affected leg; put that foot on your shoulder. Push your thumbs in between the two muscles noted above until you can feel the nerve. Compress the nerve and rhythmically move it distally until you feel a release. This technique, along with others to work on the nerve all the way to its terminus, can be added to the main techniques discussed above to improve your results.

Sacroiliac manipulations

Sacroiliac restrictions are often secondary to restrictions elsewhere in the body. In these cases, manipulation of the sacroiliac joints is worse than useless, since it wastes time and may even lead to further local irritation. However, we agree that such manipulation is beneficial for post-traumatic restriction of the sacrum. All sacroiliac joint restrictions interfere with pelvic dynamics and craniospinal dura mater mobility, and exhaust the PRM.

Sacral sidebending technique

The patient is in lateral decubitus position, with the side of the lower inferolateral angle of the sacrum on the table. As in the "lumbar roll" technique, you set up your inferior lever by flexing the hip on the ceiling side until you feel engagement of the ilium relative to the sacrum.

Your superior lever is engaged to the level of the sacrum by a very slight rotation of the trunk. The inferior hand rests on the inferolateral angle of the sacrum, which has descended. The superior hand rests on the iliac crest, and the trunk compresses the iliac wing *(Fig. 6-20)*.

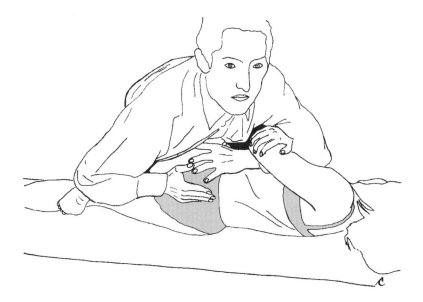

Fig. 6-20: Technique for a left sidebent sacrum

You increase traction and perform a double thrust, first in the inferior direction on the iliac crest, then superiorly under the sacral angle. You can briefly rest your chest on the iliac wing during this maneuver.

Technique for the sacrum in pseudo-rotation

This technique is similar to the preceding one.

The patient is in lateral decubitus position, on the side of the sacral pseudo-rotation. Position your inferior lever by extending the hip which is near the table. Position the superior lever by rotating the trunk to the sacrum.

Your inferior hand rests on the entire posterior hemisacrum. The forearm is perpendicular to the hand for a strictly posteroanterior thrust. Your superior arm controls the trunk at two levels: by the forearm resting on the chest, and by the hand controlling the lower lumbar area *(Fig. 6-21)*.

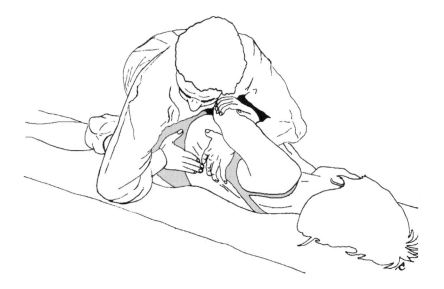

Fig. 6-21: Technique for a sacrum in pseudo right rotation

Your corrective maneuvers are performed with a general thrust together with a posteroanterior thrust on the hemisacrum posteriorly. This is done by increasing rotation of the trunk with the superior hand.

Visceral Manipulations

Visceral sheath of the neck

Global release of the sheath

If tests reveal a loss of sliding capacity of the visceral sheath on the cervical column, this technique helps restore tissue elasticity and mobility. It accomplishes mobilization through listening of the visceral structures in order to articulate them in the retropharyngoesophageal space.

As in the three-fingered test *(Fig. 5-49* in Chapter 5) of the sheath, the patient is supine, and you stand at the head. Approach the visceral sheath symmetrically at the level of the retropharyngeal and retroesophageal gliding spaces. Place your index finger on the lower part of the neck, immediately above the clavicle, your middle finger on the middle part, and your little finger on the upper part just behind the gonion *(Fig. 6-22)*.

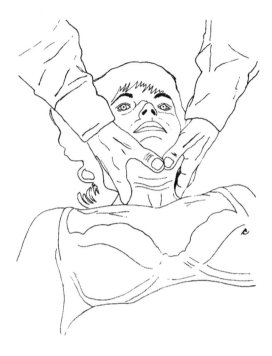

Fig. 6-22: Global technique for normalizing the visceral sheath of the neck

In the initial step, draw all the neck viscera in transverse and longitudinal mobility until you obtain a sensation of relaxation of the tissues under your fingers.

In the second step for stretching, bring the neck viscera toward the area of restricted mobility, trying to progressively improve the movement. Repeat this rhythmically four to five times until you feel a release.

Tissue restrictions of the neck are particularly anxiety-producing (inducing fear of strangulation). Be careful to follow the tissue listening during your maneuvers. Respecting the rhythm of the tissues increases tolerance for these manipulations.

Release of the prevertebral lamina of cervical fascia

If the test reveals a loss of elasticity in the prevertebral lamina (*Fig. 5-49* and text in Chapter 5), you can use a combined stretching technique which we developed with our friend and colleague Serge Levèque several years ago.

Stand on the side opposite the restricted lamina. With the tips of the fingers of your inferior hand (right hand in this illustration), work the visceral sheath in the prevertebral area of gliding, drawing the sternocleidomastoid muscle anteriorly. Delicately rotate the visceral sheath toward you. Place your superior (left) hand on the frontal to rotate the head away from you. Increase your rotation until you reach the limit of tissue elasticity, a little more with each maneuver *(Fig. 6-23)*.

After several repetitions of stretching, apply a recoil technique by abruptly but carefully releasing the support of your frontal hand at the edge of the tissue elasticity (be alert for autonomic or tension-related reactions). In this way, you produce a vibrational wave in the support system which helps restore elasticity to the tissues.

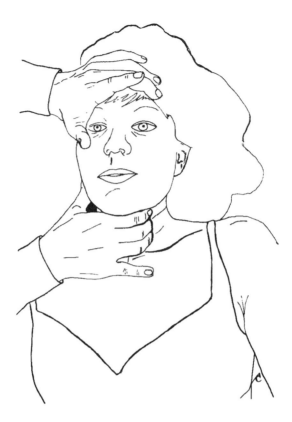

Fig. 6-23: Specific release of the prevertebral lamina of cervical fascia

Other cervical structures

This section covers the long muscle of the neck, vertebral arteries, and cervical sympathetic chain. These are not "visceral" structures per se, but may benefit from specific stretching techniques.

Stretching the long muscle of the neck

FUNCTIONAL ANATOMY

The long muscle of the neck (longus colli) is the deepest of the paravertebral muscles and plays an important role in posture and statics of the cervicothoracic spine. It extends along the anterior surface of the spinal column from the anterior arc of C1 until T3, and is comprised of three parts (inferior oblique, superior oblique, and vertical) which cover the anterior surface of the cervical spine on both sides of the median line. Bilateral, symmetric contraction of the longus colli decreases cervical lordosis and flexes the neck on the chest. Its unilateral contraction causes sidebending of the cervical spine.

The technique below is particularly effective for early sequelae of cervical trauma. A reactive spasm of this muscle is often responsible for post-traumatic cervical rigidity. We have seen many x-ray pictures revealing reversal of cervical curvature following trauma.

TECHNIQUE

Sit at the head of the supine patient. This is a unilateral technique.

With one hand, hold the patient's head above the surface of the table and braced against your chest. Keep a comfortable position, with the cervical spine straight and slightly flexed on the thorax.

Hold the cervicothoracic junction with the palm and fingers of your other hand. With your thumb, locate the anterior tubercles of the cervical transverse processes, then delicately probe along the frontal plane immediately in front of the transverse plane. Continue until you feel the indented mass of the muscle *(Fig. 6-24)*.

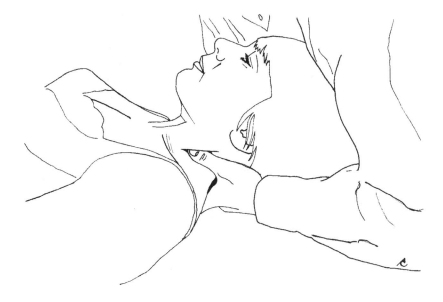

Fig. 6-24: Technique for normalizing the long muscle of the neck

Begin by directly inhibiting the muscle with the pad of your thumb, then perform stretching/listening to relax the different parts of the muscle. The stretching is done by progressively increasing the lordosis and sidebending. When the muscle is totally relaxed, rest the head and cervical spine on the table.

Stretching the vertebral arteries

These arteries play an essential role in cerebellar circulation, so their flow must remain constant, regular, and strong. The stretching technique below improves blood flow in these arteries, and also has a beneficial effect on related organs.

FUNCTIONAL ANATOMY

After C2, the vertebral artery runs to the transverse foramen of the atlas, forming a vertical concave curve inside. After exiting this foramen, it circumvents the posterior part of the lateral atlas from the outside to the inside, and also in a second horizontal and concave curve anteriorly. It then traverses the dura mater between the posterior arc of the atlas and the foramen magnum, enters the skull, circumvents the anterolateral part of the medulla oblongata, and then merges with its counterpart artery to form the basilar trunk.

The key functional areas are the transverse foramen, transverse processes of C2 and C3, and the occipitoatlantoid junction.

TECHNIQUE

The patient is supine, arms at the sides or resting on the chest. For the left vertebral artery, sit behind the patient and place your right palm or index finger under the occiput *(Fig. 6-25)*. The palm of your left hand is anterior and to the right of C7/T1, and your left thumb directed posteromedially in the direction of the cervical spine. Your left hand pushes inferiorly in addition to providing a counterforce. Your right hand draws the cervical spine in right sidebending, while maintaining the head in flexion and left rotation. Right sidebending separates the left transverse processes. It permits traction on the bends of the vertebral artery located between C2-C3 and C1-occiput.

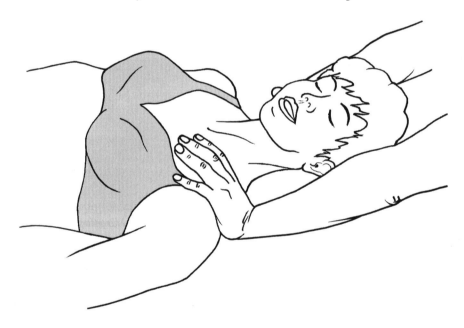

Fig. 6-25: Vertebral artery stretch

With your hands in this position, wait for the expansion phase of the PRM and stretch the occiput with your right hand. Following the listening and using real force, you encourage the stretching. The motion must be smooth and respect the orientation of the tissues. When the PRM goes into its relaxation phase, relax your pressure. Repeat until you feel a release. This technique allows for a release of both the beginning of the vertebral artery, where it branches off from the subclavian, and its end around the foramen magnum and inside the posterior fossa. The cephalad focus is on the fibers that connect the dura mater with the artery.

For treating the right vertebral artery, your left palm is under the occiput, while your right palm is anterior and to the right of C7/T1. The subsequent technique is a mirror image of that above.

INDICATIONS

This technique is useful for vertebrobasilar circulatory insufficiency, which can cause dizziness, instability, loss of balance, and problems with memory and hearing. It is also used for headaches of posterior origin. We have found this to be useful in the treatment of tinnitus, which also usually requires the treatment of the ipsilateral kidney.

With Doppler imaging, we have demonstrated improvement in basilar artery circulation by up to 30% following this technique. Disappearance of vertebrobasilar symptoms after use also proves its efficacy.

Stretching the sympathetic cervical chain

This sympathetic chain and its major superior and inferior ganglia can be treated by the technique described below.

FUNCTIONAL ANATOMY

At the cervical level, the sympathetic cord is posterior to the internal jugular vein and slightly lateral to the vagus, internal carotid, and common carotid. The cord lies against the deep cervical aponeurosis in front of the transverse processes of the cervical vertebrae, from which it is separated by the long muscle of the neck (see above) and rectus capitis anterior.

The superior cervical ganglion is the largest (2-4cm). It lies on each side of the pharynx in front of C2-C3, rests posteriorly on the rectus capitis anterior, and is covered by the deep cervical aponeurosis (Fig. 6-26).

The deep cervical aponeurosis is attached superiorly to the basilar part of the occiput by exchange of fibers with the dura mater, and laterally to the cervical transverse processes where it is continued by the aponeurosis of the anterior scalene. Inferiorly, at the level of the upper thoracic vertebrae, it joins to the cellular tissue of the posterior mediastinum.

The inferior cervical ganglion is in front of the transverse process of C7, behind the point of origin of the vertebral artery.

TECHNIQUE

This technique is not specific to the sympathetic cervical chain. It also affects the cervical spine and associated muscles, aponeuroses, and cervicopleural attachments, and decreases the general tone of the sympathetic nervous system.

The patient is supine, cervical spine slightly extended. For stretching the right sympathetic chain, the nape of the neck rests on your right palm. The palm of your left hand is placed behind the clavicle in the direction of the first rib approximately 1.5cm from the sternoclavicular joint toward the scalene tubercle of Lisfranc. For stretching the left sympathetic chain, the position of your hands is reversed.

Stretch the nape of the neck in rotation and sidebending while supporting the first rib and clavicle, or pushing them inferolaterally to emphasize the stretching. Stretching takes place through the aponeurosis of the long muscle of the neck, which has a direct relation with the sympathetic cervical chain. Reflex improvement in vertebral artery circulation is obtained from the mechanical action on the sympathetic chain.

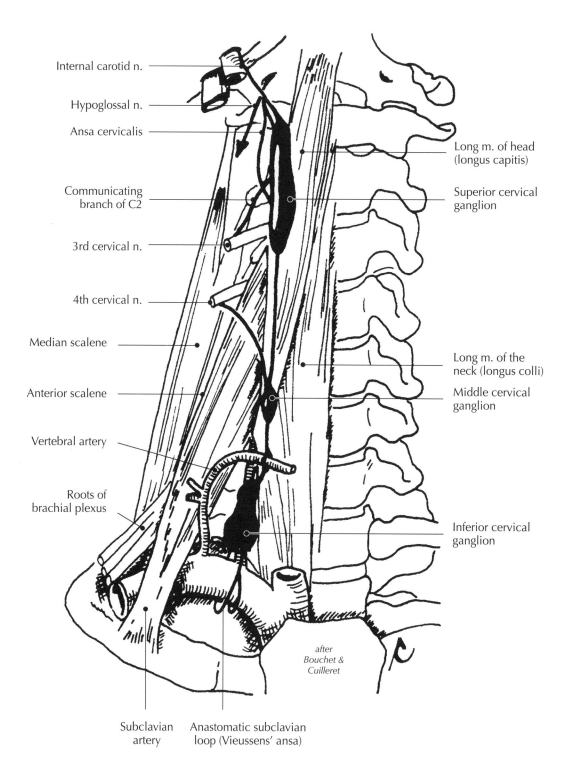

Internal carotid n.

Hypoglossal n.

Ansa cervicalis

Communicating
branch of C2

3rd cervical n.

4th cervical n.

Median scalene

Anterior scalene

Vertebral artery

Roots of
brachial plexus

Long m. of head
(longus capitis)

Superior cervical
ganglion

Long m. of the
neck (longus colli)

Middle cervical
ganglion

Inferior cervical
ganglion

*after
Bouchet &
Cuilleret*

Subclavian
artery

Anastomatic subclavian
loop (Vieussens' ansa)

Fig. 6-26: Cervical sympathetic chain

Left kidney

Supine position

The patient is supine, arms resting on the chest, left leg flexed. Standing and facing the patient's left side, place the radial edge of your right index finger between the iliac crest and left twelfth rib, and your thumb on the lateral corresponding part of the descending colon. Your right elbow is flexed and pressed against your hip for better support. Your left palm is against the inferior pole of the left kidney, located deep to the duodenojejunal junction *(Fig. 6-27)*.

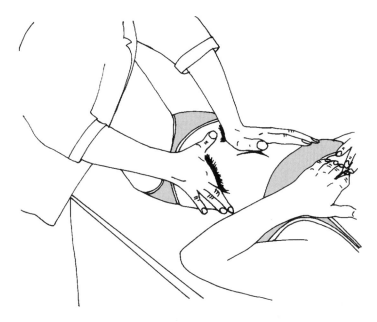

Fig. 6-27: Manipulation of the left kidney: supine position

Direct technique

Use both hands to push the kidney anteriorly, superiorly, and medially. The right index finger together with the other fingers first push the kidney anteriorly. The left palm can then be better positioned against the inferior pole, and both hands work together to push the kidney medially and superiorly.

The criterion of success is when the right index finger, located in Grynfelt's triangle, can move with ease. Grynfelt's triangle becomes more easily depressible and less sensitive to probing. At the end of the manipulation, probing should be painless.

Indirect technique

The right index finger and left palm first find their direction before slightly relaxing the pressure and following the direction of listening. The movement is a rather pronounced induction, and you follow the movement of listening with the same force used for the direct technique.

Right lateral decubitus position

FIRST METHOD

The patient lies on the right side, right leg extended, left leg flexed, head on a cushion or the flexed right forearm. Place your right thumb in Grynfelt's triangle and your right palm against the posteromedial part of the iliac crest. Your left palm exerts counterforce on the left costochondral joints *(Fig. 6-28)*.

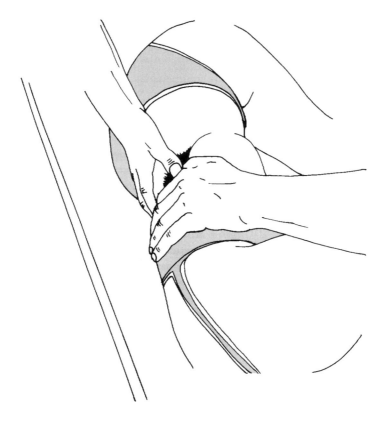

Fig. 6-28: Manipulation of the left kidney: right lateral decubitus position (1st method)

Direct technique

Push your right thumb anteriorly, medially, and superiorly to mobilize the left kidney. With your left hand, mobilize the left rib cage, from outside to inside, to facilitate contact of right thumb with the kidney. With a major renal restriction, you may feel a crackling of neighboring tissues while mobilizing the kidney due to fibrosis of perirenal fat.

Indirect technique

After directly mobilizing the kidney as above, we use the indirect technique to release a restricted attachment or fascia located deep in the back. The kidney itself does not have linear mobility. In the event of ptosis, indirect techniques give better mobilization and repositioning. Always act in the direction of the repositioning.

SECOND METHOD

Stand behind the patient, who is in right lateral decubitus position, as above. Place your right thumb in Grynfelt's triangle, and the rest of your hand against the latissimus dorsi and paravertebral musculature. Brace your elbow against your right hip to increase the force of penetration by your right thumb. Your left hand, positioned against the left costochondral joints, pushes them posteriorly and outward. To mobilize the kidney properly, your thumb should be directed anteriorly, medially, and superiorly (Fig. 6-29).

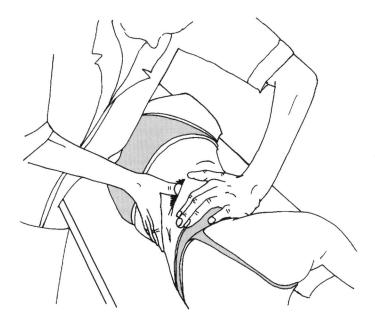

Fig. 6-29: Manipulation of the left kidney: right lateral decubitus position (2nd method)

Use the indirect technique at the end of the movement. The maneuver is complete when your fingers no longer encounter resistance, and the sensitivity or pain in Grynfelt's triangle has disappeared. With practice, this difference will be obvious.

Technique using the left leg

The patient is supine, arms on the chest, left leg flexed. Facing the patient's left side, place the radial edge of your right index finger in the left Grynfelt's triangle. With your left hand, grasp the left knee and draw it in abduction and flexion. This relaxes the myofascial structures of Grynfelt's triangle, facilitating the penetration of your right index finger and making it easier to find the restricted tissues and to press behind the inferior pole of the kidney (Fig. 6-30).

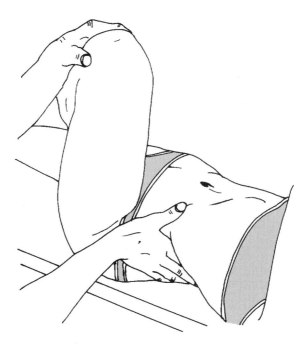

Fig. 6-30: Combined manipulation of the left kidney and leg

Maintain the pressure of your right index finger. Mobilize the knee, bringing the left leg in internal rotation, adduction, and extension, until the leg rests on the table.

This powerful technique is used for significant restrictions of the kidney in which the perirenal tissues have undergone fibrosis. It requires good coordination but can produce great improvement in symptoms.

Spleen

The first step in manual treatment of the spleen is to release the ligaments, omentum, and fascia which link it to the neighboring organs, diaphragm, and skeleton. Next, you mobilize it in its compartment.

Gastrophrenic ligament

The patient is seated, arms resting on the thighs. Standing behind the patient, use your left palm to push the anterolateral part of the left rib cage medially and anteriorly so as to more easily access the deep elements of the gastrophrenic ligament. Your left fingers are directed toward the ligament *(Fig. 6-31)*. Starting from the lateral edge of the rectus, direct the fingers of your right hand superiorly, posteriorly, and slightly medially until they meet the attachment of the greater curvature on the diaphragm and its extensions toward the left phrenicocolic ligament.

Problems with the spleen usually involve the posterolateral portion of the gastrophrenic ligament. Directly release the support tissues by stretching them anterolaterally, then raise the external part of the stomach several times to relax its attachments.

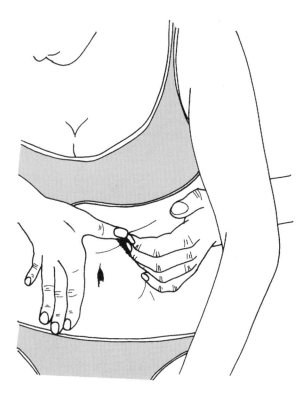

Fig. 6-31: Manipulation of the gastrophrenic ligament

Indirect techniques are recommended for the gastrophrenic ligament, which is rich in mechanoreceptors. After you have relaxed the tissues, mobilize the patient's chest in flexion and right sidebending. Then reassume your initial position and begin again.

When your fingers are on a stretched area, maintain their pressure and use manipulation/stretching of the thorax to release ligamentous/fascial tensions. Move the patient's body around the restrictions, instead of applying the force of your hands directly to the restricted areas. This is less irritating and uncomfortable for the patient, and is also more effective.

Transverse mesocolon

This is often neglected by osteopaths, but is important for treatment of the spleen—in particular, its attachments on the posterior parietal peritoneum and its extensions toward the left phrenicocolic ligament and spleen.

The patient is supine, arms at the sides, legs flexed. Stand behind the patient's head or left shoulder, and place your two thumbs over the splenic and hepatic flexures of the colon (summits of the descending and ascending colons respectively). With your hands flattened against the left and right flanks, direct your thumbs medially, posteriorly, and inferiorly *(Fig. 6-32)*. Slightly relax the pressure, and follow the direction of listening.

We prefer manipulating the transverse mesocolon in the supine position, because this facilitates relaxation of the muscular/ligamentous/fascial system of the abdomen.

Our goal is not only to release restricted fibers, but also to deeply manipulate the affected tissues. For similar reasons, we find indirect listening-based techniques more effective here than direct techniques.

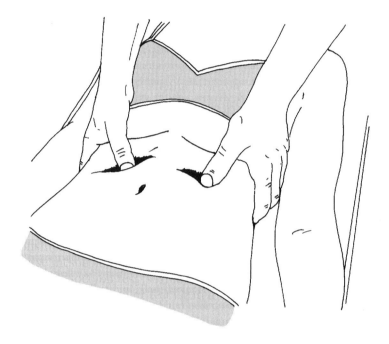

Fig. 6-32: Manipulation of the transverse mesocolon: supine position

Left phrenicocolic ligament

The patient is seated, hands on the thighs. Stand behind the patient, with your right knee on the table to stabilize yourself. Place your left hand against the left rib cage and the fingers of your right hand below the rib cage, in an anterolateral position *(Fig. 6-33)*. Bring the left rib cage anteriorly, medially, and inferiorly. Take advantage of the relaxation of abdominal tissues to stretch the fibers of the phrenicocolic ligament with your right hand.

First, stretch the fibers which are directed toward the stomach, then those which run toward the transverse mesocolon, and finally those which run to the diaphragm. Mobilize the splenic flexure of the colon several times and repeat the procedure until all the attachments have been relaxed.

For a restriction which seems significant, leave your fingers *in situ* by lightly manipulating the stretched fibers in the direction of listening, and move the patient's thorax around this region. This is an excellent method for painlessly releasing the phrenicocolic attachments of the spleen.

Mobilization of the splenic attachments

The patient's position is the same as above. Again, place your fingers as deeply and high as possible in the anterolateral position under the rib cage. Draw the thorax in left rotation and extension, while raising the left phrenicocolic region.

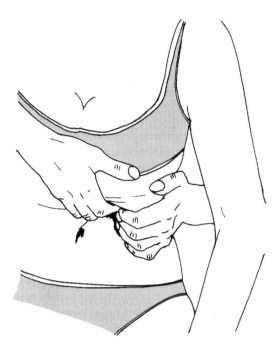

Fig. 6-33: Manipulation of the left phrenicocolic ligament: seated position

Perform this movement three or four times with the direct technique, then mobilize the thorax and subcostal fingers in the direction of listening. When properly executed, this maneuver should not cause pain.

Left triangular ligament of the liver

The patient's position is the same as above. With your right knee on the table, place your left palm on the anterior left rib cage, at the level of the eighth through tenth costochondral joints, so that your fingers are 5 or 6cm below the costal margin (*Fig. 6-34*).

DIRECT TECHNIQUE

Place your right fingers on the linea alba. The fingers of both hands are directed posteriorly, superiorly, and to the left. Your left palm draws the ribs anteriorly, medially, and inferiorly. Place the right fingers against the left edge of the liver, and you should feel the left triangular ligament as a fibrous lamina with harder consistency than that of neighboring tissues. Mobilize this lamina posteriorly and anteriorly, taking care not to cause pain.

INDIRECT TECHNIQUE

Your position and the placement of your hands are the same as for the direct technique above. From this position, focusing on the structure of the left triangular ligament, you follow the listening. This essential technique permits your hands to go directly to

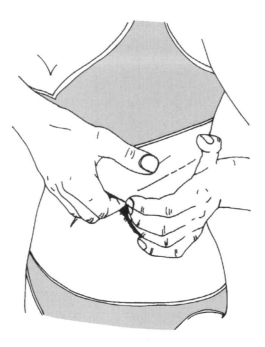

Fig. 6-34: Manipulation of the left triangular ligament

the restriction while also mobilizing the thorax in the direction of listening. The left triangular ligament is rich in proprioceptors, and relaxing it provides an important release for the surrounding ligamentous/fascial and corresponding osteoarticular system.

Ribs in relation to the spleen

The patient is supine, arms crossed on the chest, legs extended. Standing to the right, position your right hand under the eighth through tenth left ribs, with your fingertips on the posterior angles. The left hand is placed on the thorax as a counterforce. Draw the ribs anteriorly, medially, and slightly inferiorly.

This technique should follow other subthoracic visceral manipulations. To obtain best results on the spleen, draw the ribs in the direction of listening. At the end of treatment, the impression of restricted mobilization should be gone.

Vertebrae

We are not describing vertebral manipulations in this book, but will make a few general comments.

It is very rare to find a post-traumatic splenic restriction that is not accompanied by vertebral or costovertebral restriction of T8-10. We routinely release the soft perisplenic tissues prior to osteoarticular manipulation, since this gives better and more lasting results.

Likewise, restrictions of the first rib are usually secondary to a problem elsewhere, so we always seek out the viscera or attachments responsible for underlying mechanical tension. Since the first rib is most often secondary, if we perform direct manipulation, especially the high-velocity type, there is a risk of provoking cervicobra-chial neuralgia.

The first lumbar vertebra is often involved in post-traumatic splenic restrictions. This vertebra plays the role of "overflow" for the body, and its restrictions are rarely attributable to a specific organ. We often manipulate it because it permits us to obtain a good diaphragmatic release.

Motility of the liver, spleen, and kidney

Every day, trauma specialists diagnose ruptures of these three solid organs, which are vulnerable to impact of all types. These ruptures cannot be taken lightly, and can even be fatal.

"Who is capable of the most is capable of the least!" is an adage difficult to prove. However, if visceral rupture results from severe trauma, it seems likely that less severe trauma may also affect these organs.

In clinical practice, we frequently find restrictions of these organs following tissue trauma. It is important to return mobility without neglecting motility. Restitution of motility is what restores, to these organs and the patient, the energy which is lacking after trauma. This is the "extra" supplied by osteopathy in comparison to conventional medicine.

Chapter Seven:
Conclusion

We hope that this book has conveyed to our readers the power and specificity of the osteopathic approach to trauma. Some other important aspects of our approach include the following.

It is global.

All macro- or micro-elements of the human body can be injured by the forces of collision, causing local or general disequilibrium. A psychoemotional component must also be considered, which is capable of greatly increasing tissue restrictions, or even creating them.

It searches for the cause.

The symptoms are part of the osteopathic diagnosis which we take into account, but without regarding them as being the major cause of mechanical restriction. We always try to find the cause of tissue restrictions, which often have no obvious relationship to the symptoms manifested.

It involves the tissues.

The tissues possess an infallible memory for trauma. Everything is recorded in them. Each tissue in the human body is worthy of interest and contributes to a person's history.

It is manual.

In osteopathy, both diagnosis and treatment are done with the hands.

It is subtle.

A certain progression of testing and evaluation is essential to demonstrate the unexpected effects of traumatic sequelae, particularly if the injury is an old one.

It is filled with respect.

Brute force is never one of the osteopath's tools. Tissues can only be treated if the osteopath respects them. The right key can easily unlock the door.

It is both scientific and empirical.

Osteopathy requires much knowledge and training, but none of us can deny the empirical aspect which is an integral part of our special art and science.

Painting is based on three primary colors, combined in an infinite number of nuances. Each painter uses them in an individual way, according to his or her inspiration. Music is based on a mere twelve notes, but their arrangement and combinations are infinite. Osteopathy is based upon elements of anatomy, medical science, and human mechanics, but developed and applied in unique and varied ways. Our field is different from allopathic medicine but complementary, for the ultimate benefit of the patient.

Even though osteopathy is a unified discipline in its fundamental concepts, each of its interpreters is an individual. Using the same colors and notes, each practitioner has free rein to express his or her inspiration to find new or more effective ways to improve the patient's physical and emotional well-being.

Bibliography

Anselmet P. "Analysis of lesions of the thorax and abdomen in automobile accident victims." *Theses in Medicine*, 1985.

Arlot J. *Notes personnelles.* Grenoble: Revol, 1991.

Barral JP. *The Thorax.* Seattle: Eastland Press, 1991.

Barral JP. *Urogenital Manipulation.* Seattle: Eastland Press, 1993.

Barral JP. *Manual Thermal Diagnosis.* Seattle: Eastland Press, 1996.

Barral JP. *Visceral Manipulation II.* Seattle: Eastland Press, 1989.

Barral JP, Ligner B, Paoletti S, Prat D, Rommeveaux L, Triana D. *Nouvelles techniques uro-génitales.* Aix en Provence: Cido & De Verlaque Editions, 1993.

Barral JP, Mathieu JP, Mercier P. *Diagnostic articulaire vertébral.* Aix en Provence: Cido & De Verlaque Editions, 1992.

Barral JP, Mercier P. *Visceral Manipulation.* Seattle: Eastland Press, 1988.

Becker RE. "Whiplash Injuries." *Academy of Applied Osteopathy Yearbook of Selected Osteopathic Papers*, 1958.

Becker RE. "Whiplash Injury." *Academy of Applied Osteopathy Yearbook of Selected Osteopathic Papers*, 1964.

Borgi R, Plas F. *Traumatologie et rééducation*. Paris: Masson, 1982.

Bouchet Y, Cuilleret J. *Anatomie topographique, fonctionnelle et descriptive*. Lyon: Simep, 1983.

Bourg M. *"Eléments de Mécanique"* in Poitout D. *Biomécanique Orthopédique*. Paris: Masson, 1987.

Bozetto M. *Lésions et corrections crâiniennes*. Nice: ATMAN, 1982.

Breig A. *Adverse Mechanical Tension in the Central Nervous System*. New York: John Wiley and Sons, 1978.

Brizon J, Castaing J. *Les Feuillets d'Anatomie. Volume 14: le Thorax*. Paris: Maloine, 1953.

Camirand N, Muzzi D. *"Influence de la liberation du core-link sur le tonus musculaire paravertebral."* Unpublished thesis, College Osteopathique du Montreal, 1993.

Carpenter MB. *Human Neuroanatomy*. Baltimore: Williams & Wilkins, 1976.

Castaing J. *Anatomie fonctionnelle de l'appareil locomoteur*. Paris: Vigot, 1960.

Cerisier P. *"Notion de Résistance des Matériaux"* in Poitout D. *Biomécanique Orthopédique*. Paris: Masson, 1987.

Chaillet AH. *Histoire du liquide céphalo-rachidien*. Lyon: Thèse Médecine, 1985.

Chapon A. "Human tolerance to impact and possible method for an improvement in knowledge." *Rapport ONSER*, 1978.

Croibier A. *Trou obturateur, énigme ostéopathique*. Unpublished thesis, 1991.

Cuzin E. Personal communication, 1992.

Delmas A. *Voies et centres nerveux*. Paris: Masson, 1973.

Doury P. *Algosystrophies: Clinque et Diagnostique*. Paris: Laboratoires Armour Montagu, 1984.

Fink BR, Walker S. "Orientation of the fibers in human dorsal lumbar dura mater in relation to lumbar puncture." *Anesthesia Analgesia* 1985, 69(6):768-72.

Frymann V. Personal communication, 1996.

Fryette HH. *Principles of Osteopathic Technic*. Carmel, CA: Academy of Applied Osteopathy, 1954.

Gabarel B, Roques M. *Les Fasciae en médecine ostéopathique*. Paris: Maloine, 1985.

Goldsmith W. "The physical processes producing heat injuries" in Caveness W. F. and Walker AE. *Head Injury Conference Procedings*. Philadelphia: J. B. Lippincott, 1966, 350-82.

Gordon JE. *Structures et matériaux. L'explication mécanique des formes. Pour la science*. Belin diffusion, 1994.

Guerit JM. *"Les comas"* in *La recherche* 1990, 21:1026-36.

Gurdjian ES, Webster JE, *Head Injuries: Mechanisms, Diagnosis, and Management*. Boston: Little, Brown, 1958.

Haines DE. "On the question of the subdural space." *Anat. Rec.*, 1990, 230(1):3-21.

Harakal J. H. "An osteopathically integrated approach to the whiplash complex." *JAOA* 1975, 74(6):59-74.

Hardy A. *Introduction à l'ostéopathie crânienne ; le dommage du coup de fouet, whiplash injury son diagnostic, sa thérapeutique*. Paris: Peyronnet, 1967.

Heilig D. "Whiplash mechanics of injury: management of cervical and dorsal involvement." *JAOA* 1963, 10:52-59.

Hugues FC. *Pathologie respiratoire*. Paris: Heures de France, 1971.

Iyer RP, "Seat-belt syncope." *The Lancet* 1995: 346, 1044.

Issartel L, Issartel M. *L'ostéopathie exactement*. Paris: Robert Laffont, 1983.

Kahle W, Leonhardt H, Platzer W. *Anatomie*. Paris: Flammarion, 1979.

Kamina P. *Anatomie gynécologique et obstétricale*. Paris: Maloine, 1984.

Kane J, Sternheim M. *Physics*. Paris: InterEditions, 1986.

Korr I. *The Neurobiologic Mechanisms in Manipulative Therapy*. New York: Plenum, 1978.

Laborit H. *L'Inhibition de l'action: Biologie, physiologie, psychologie, sociologie*. Paris: Masson, 1981.

Lacan J. Personal communication, 1972.

La Vielle J, Roux H, Stanoyevitch JF. *Le système vertébro-basilaire*. Marseille: Sola, 1986.

Lazorthes G. *Le système nerveux périphérique.* Paris: Masson, 1971.

Lazorthes G, Poulhes J, Gaubert M. *"La dure-mère de la charnière crânio-rachidienne."* *Bull. Assoc. Anat.* 1953, 78:169-72.

Leveque S. *Contribution à l'étude des conséquences ostéopathiques des atteintes tissulaires pleuro-pulmonaires.* Unpublished thesis, 1991.

Livingston RB. "Mechanics of Cerebrospinal Fluid" in Ruch TC, Patton HD, *Physiology and Biophysics.* Philadelphia: W. B. Saunders Company, 1965: 935-40.

Louis R. *"Dynamique vertébro-radiculaire et vertébro-médullaire."* *Anat. Clin.* 1981, 3: 1-11.

Lucas P, Stehman M. "Étude sur la proprioception." Free University of Brussels, 1992.

Magoun HI. *Osteopathy in the Cranial Field.* Kirksville, MO: The Journal Printing Company, 1966.

Magoun HI. "Whiplash injury: a greater lesion complex." *Academy of Applied Osteopathy Yearbook of Selected Osteopathic Papers*, 1976.

Maideu J. Presentation at the American Academy of Neurology, 1991.

Maillot C. *"Les espaces périmédullaires. Constitution, organisation et relations avec le liquide cérébro-spinal."* *J. Neuroradiol.* 1990: 71, 10:539-47.

Manelfe C. *Imagerie du rachis et de la moelle.* Paris: Vigot, 1989.

Mathieu JP, Mercier P, Barral JP. *Diagnostic articulaire vertébral, 2° édition.* Aix en Provence: Editions Cido & De Verlaque, 1992.

Mitchell FL, Moran PS, Pruzzo NA. *An Evaluation and Treatment Manual of Osteopathic Muscle Energy Procedures.* Valley Park, MO: Institute for Continuing Education in Osteopathic Principles, 1979.

Mnidiru J. Presentation, American Academy of Neurology, 1991.

Mohr B. *"Apport de l'imagerie conventionnelle en ostéopathie."* Personal notes, Metz, 1997.

Olivier G. *Anatomie Anthropologique.* Paris: Vigot, 1965.

Oosterveld WJ. *"Le appareil vestibulaire et cellule ciliée."* *Impact Médicine*, 1991, 105:5.

Papassin JJ. *Le Médiastin organe ostéopathique.* Grenoble: Editions des sources, 1991.

Patel A, et al. *Abrégé de traumatologie*. Paris: Masson, 1988.

Paturet G. *Traité d'anatomie humaine*. Paris: Masson, 1951.

DePeretti F, Micalef JP, Bourgeon A, Argenson C, Rabischong P. "Biomechanics of the lumbar spinal nerve roots and the first sacral root within the intervertebral foramina." *Surg. Radiol. Anat.* 1989, 11(3):221-22.

Perlemuter L, Waligora J. *Cahiers d'anatomie*. Paris: Masson, 1975.

Pialot V. *"Les mécanismes de l'éveil"* in *Science et Vie* 1996, 195:62-68.

Pouilhe G. *La dure-mère rachidienne*. Unpublished thesis, 1994.

Prat D. *Notes personnelles*. Bourgoin: Editions de La Grive, 1992.

Rabischong P. *"Anatomie fonctionnelle du rachis et de la moelle"* in Manelfe C. *Imagerie du rachis et de la moelle*. Paris: Vigot, 1989.

Richard JP. *La colonne vertébrale en ostéopathie*. Aix en Provence: De Verlaque Editions, 1987.

Rommeveaux L. *Notes personnelles*. Grenoble: Editions de La Charmette, 1993.

Rouviere H. *Anatomie humaine descriptive et topographique*. Paris: Masson, 1948.

Schuller E. *"Liquide céphalorachidien"* in *Encycl. Méd. Chir. — Neurologie*. Paris: Editions Techniques. 1993.

Povlishock JT, Becker DP, Cheng CL, Vaughan GW. "Axonal changes in minor head injury." *J Neuropathol. Exp. Neurol.* 1983, 42:223-42.

Strachan WF. "Applied anatomy of the pelvis and perineum." *JAOA* 1939, 38:8.

Sutherland WG. *Teachings in the Science of Osteopathy*. Ed. by Anne Wales. Portland, OR: Rudra Press, 1990.

Swierzewski MJ, Feliciano DV, Lillis RP, Illig KA, States JD. "Deaths from motor vehicle crashes: patterns of injury in restrained and unrestrained victims." *Journal of Trauma* 1994, 37(3):404-7.

Testut L. *Traité d'anatomie humaine*. Paris: Octave Doin, 1889.

Testut L, Jacob O. *Anatomie topographique*. Paris: Gaston Doin, 1927.

Trias A. "Effect of persistent pressure on the articular cartilage: an experimental study."*Journal of Bone Joint Surgery* (Br) 1961, 43:376-86.

Tricot P. *L'ostéopathie, une technique pour libérer la vie.* Paris: Chiron, 1992.

Upledger JE, Vredevoogd JD. *Craniosacral Therapy.* Chicago: Eastland Press, 1983.

Verriest JP, et al. *"La tolérance humaine aux chocs" INRETS.* Recherche Transports et Sécurité, June 1986.

Williams N, Leveau B, Lissner HR. *Biomechanics of Human Motion.* Philadelphia: W. B. Saunders Company, 1977.

Williams P, Warwick R, eds. *Gray's Anatomy.* Edinburgh: Livingstone, 1980.

Wright JM. "Whiplash injuries: management and complications." *JAOA* 1956, 55:564-66.

Wright S. et al. *Physiologie appliquée à la médecine.* Paris: Flammarion Médicine-Sciences, 1973.

List of Illustrations

CHAPTER ONE

CHAPTER TWO

CHAPTER THREE

CHAPTER FOUR

CHAPTER FIVE

CHAPTER SIX

Index